T0277438

Kosher Lust

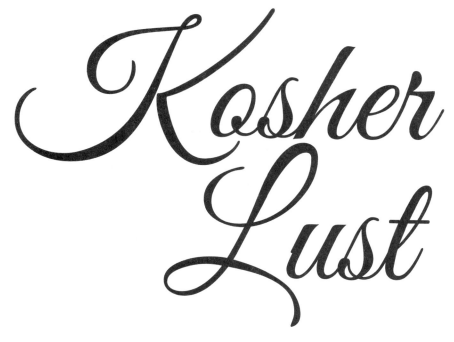

Love is NOT the Answer

RABBI SHMULEY BOTEACH

International Bestselling Author of *Kosher Sex*

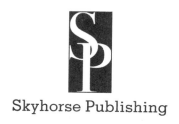

Skyhorse Publishing

Skyhorse Publishing books may be purchased in bulk at special discounts for sales promotion, corporate gifts, fund-raising, or educational purposes. Special editions can also be created to specifications. For details, contact the Special Sales Department, Skyhorse Publishing, 307 West 36th Street, 11th Floor, New York, NY 10018 or info@skyhorsepublishing.com.

Skyhorse® and Skyhorse Publishing® are registered trademarks of Skyhorse Publishing, Inc.®, a Delaware corporation.

Visit our website at www.skyhorsepublishing.com.
Please follow our publisher Tony Lyons on Instagram @tonylyonsisuncertain

10 9 8 7 6 5 4 3 2 1

Library of Congress Cataloging-in-Publication Data is available on file.

Print ISBN: 978-1-5107-7995-2
eBook ISBN: 978-1-5107-7996-9

Cover design by David Ter-Avanesyan

Printed in the United States of America

DEDICATION

To Miriam and Sheldon

for your love of America,
total devotion to the Jewish people,
and unwavering support of Israel

and, most importantly,

for the example you set
for what a married couple can accomplish together
in making the world a better place

Contents

Preface · ix

PART 1

Unavailability: The Loss of Lust in Our Lives

CHAPTER 1 Love Won't Keep Us Together · 3
  Love: The Downfall of the American Marriage · 3
  A Force Much Stronger Than Love · 8
  The Core Issue · 10

CHAPTER 2 The Sexually Extinguished Wife · 18
  A Woman's Primary Need · 18
  The *Fifty Shades of Grey* Phenomenon · 31
  The Grand Extinguisher · 37

CHAPTER 3 What Men Are Looking For · 52
  Not Good for Man to Be Alone · 52
  Why Men Look Elsewhere · 59
  Tuning In · 68

PART 2

Mystery: What We Need to Know about Lust

CHAPTER 4 What Is This Thing Called Lust? · 81
  A Definition · 81
  The Three Principles of Lust · 90
  Is There Hope for Lust in Marriage? · 99

CHAPTER 5 The Unappreciated Treasure: Why We Shun Lust · 101
  We Believe Lust Is Transient · 101
  We Believe God Is Love and Lust Is Wrong · 107
  We Believe Lust Is Politically Incorrect · 112

CHAPTER 6 Cleaving: Love and Lust in the Hebrew
Bible · 118

The Holy of Holies · 118
Devekut – Cleaving · 126
Biblical Marriages · 130

**PART 3
Sinfulness: Getting to Forbidden Territory**

CHAPTER 7 Vive la Différence: Magnetizing Marriage · 139

Keep Your Distance · 139
Curb TMI · 148
Get into Mischief · 153

CHAPTER 8 The Paradox of Trust · 161

The Essential Contradiction · 161
The Positive Power of Jealousy · 168
Going Deeper with Trust · 174

CHAPTER 9 Flesh of My Flesh: A Return to Eden · 182

The Goal-Oriented Approach · 182
Physical and Spiritual Transcendence · 191
A Working Model · 204

Acknowledgments · 215

Notes · 217

Preface

What happened to love? It seems to have a short shelf life these days. People fall in love and expect to be happy but find themselves a little while later not as excited and not as engaged. I meet couples like this nearly every day: their marriages feel boring and stultifying, their relationships lack passion. We all aspire to fall in love and stay in love. Yet we struggle to find examples of people who've actually found the happiness they seek.

Sure, many married couples seem stable and comfortable. But not necessarily that excited. Marriage may provide them children and permanence. But its routine doesn't give them a lot to look forward to.

This a revolutionary book. I know that an author should not say that, but I truly believe it. There are thousands of books on love and marriage, but this one is different. It does not try to fix love but rather argues that the problem is love itself. Love was never meant to serve as the glue that keeps couples romantically together. Love simply is not strong enough to do that.

Essentially, you've been lied to throughout your life about relationships. Every time you saw a couple in a movie fall in love and then – fast forward – marrying and living happily ever after, you were misled. Not because that couple could not remain in love forever. Of course they could. But rather because Hollywood did not show you the "happily ever after" married couple's sex life being reduced to once a week for about ten minutes at a time.

In other words, they did not show you the couple gradually losing the passionate adhesive that kept them longing for each other.

The principal reason for the breakdown of marriages and relationships is that in modern times they are built not on lust but on love. That's right: *love has been a disappointment.* It's simply not strong enough to keep a man and a woman excited about each other over the decades.

But lust is.

Lust, the most powerful force in the universe, is the real glue between a man and a woman, and in this book I'm going to prove to you that marriages are meant to be based on lust, and not just on love. Furthermore, I'm going to prove to you that contrary to popular wisdom, lust does not have to fade away. It can – and must – be maintained over the long term, for without it, marriages are destined to wither.

In our day, women especially are suffering the loss of lust. They feel loved but not desired, cherished but not yearned for, which is why, even more than men, they are becoming disillusioned with marriage and relationships.

Several times a week I counsel couples in crisis. They come with the usual panoply of issues that surround broken marriages: an absence of communication, lack of intimacy, fighting below the belt, financial pressures, and responsibilities of child rearing that have overtaken their lives.

But underlying all these problems is the elephant in the room: a loss of desire. They love each other, but they no longer hunger and thirst for each other. Their marriages are now built on the softer, more comfortable emotion of love rather than on the passionate, more explosive bond of lust.

You would be hard pressed to find a single relationships expert or marital counselor anywhere who would argue that marriages should be based on lust rather than love. Indeed, they would probably say that my words in so advocating are irresponsible. The marriage counselors tell me I'm wrong and I'm raising people's expectations unfairly. But when I speak on the subject, the wives sit in their seats and their heads begin to nod approvingly as I present my material. They give their husbands knowing looks as I speak of a woman's need to be not just loved but deeply desired.

If the relationships experts are right and I'm wrong, why is marriage dying? Forget the 50 percent divorce rate that has prevailed for a half century or more.[1] I'm talking about people no longer believing in marriage but rather in serial monogamy. More and more we are hearing arguments to the effect that today's increased life span spells an end to monogamy as a way of life. People used to die at fifty, so marriages were not expected to last longer than about thirty years. Now that people live till eighty,[2] there is no way marriages should be expected to last fifty years or more. We now outlive the natural life span of a marriage, according to this view, and serial monogamy is the best we can hope for.

So people are shacking up more and marrying less. Married couples are today in the United States, for the first time ever, a minority of households.[3] Nearly half of all women are single.[4] Hollywood is famous for men and women who have children together but who never even think of marrying. Why should they? Their commitment to one another is enough. Once the commitment wears off, they'll separate amicably – or not amicably – and move on to the next person. Why remain tied in a loveless relationship? Take what you can get, for as long as you can get it, and move on.

What certainly cannot be said is that marriage is dying due to a lack of information. There are arguably more self-help books on marriage and relationships being published every year than in all of human history prior to the modern era. More relationship advice is arguably being dispensed in one day of TV than most of our grandparents received in a lifetime.

So why are relationships on the decline? Because the advice being given is flawed. It's based on love and not lust. It glorifies closeness without emphasizing distance. It promotes total familiarity and discounts mystery. It focuses on the legality of marriage rather than the sinfulness of forbidden desire. In short, it highlights the warm embers of friendship over the flaming coals of lust.

But how did we get it so wrong? How did love come to trump lust? Why have we come to base marriages on the weaker link of love instead of the nuclear bond of lust?

Lust has been lost from our lives because we think it is something lowly, a visceral emotion demonstrating more our kinship with animals than anything uniquely human. We associate it with the body rather than with the soul, believing it to be generated by hormones rather than a spiritual energy. And because we don't understand lust, we have never focused on mastering its rules and the conditions through which it is maintained.

Moreover, in a culture where almost everything a man wants from a woman he can conveniently get from porn, or from sex on a first date, it's all so open and available that there is no room for lust to develop.

Then there is this: we believe love to be eternal while lust is so utterly ephemeral. We deemphasize lust in relationships because we believe it's bound to disappoint us and let us down. We don't believe that lust can be sustained. It's a flimsy foundation upon which to build a relationship, says the common wisdom, and should be made secondary to the solid firmament of love.

But it is in fact love that has failed us, because we're asking more from love than it can reasonably give. Love is warm; lust is passionate. Love seeks to share; lust seeks to dominate and conquer. While love can be satiated, lust, practiced properly, never can.

Only lust can create the primal bond that keeps a man and a woman magnetized to each other. Only lust can truly invigorate a marriage. Indeed, as I'm going to show you in this book, the Hebrew Bible advocates lust as the basis of marriage, and the book identified by the Talmud as the holiest book in the Bible raises lust to a pinnacle of holiness.

You may be wondering, if lust is really kosher, why are people so opposed to it?

In fact, you may be thinking, isn't lust pornographic, sleazy, transient, misogynistic? Beneath us?

Love is glorious! Love is romantic, beautiful, solid.

Lust is dirty by comparison, fleeting, unreliable.

Yet I maintain that because we build marriages on a foundation of love and ignore lust, our marriages don't have nearly the spark they should and they risk becoming a bore.

In this book I'm going to challenge you to overturn your assumptions about love and lust.

You've been taught that lust is base and degrading. This is because we have denigrated lust and made it about sleaze. Lust is what men feel when they look at porn. Lust is what is created on the dance floor at a club.

That's not the lust we're talking about.

What we're discussing is kosher lust, holy lust, the kind described in the ancient Kabbalistic literature as the yearning of the soul for God, the striving of the spirit for the divine. *Ki zeh kamah nichsof nichsafti*, "Oh, how I have lusted and longed for Your glorious presence," says the Hebrew liturgical poem "Yedid Nefesh," recited every Friday evening as the Sabbath begins. Isaac Luria, the sixteenth-century father of modern Kabbalah, wrote in "Bnei Heichala," sung by many at the third meal of the Jewish Sabbath, "You princes of the palace [Torah scholars] who lust and long to behold the countenance of the Divine Presence."

The lust we're talking about is what Abraham felt for Sarah, what Isaac and Rebecca feel for each other the first time they meet, what Jacob felt for Rachel for whom he was forced to work for seven years and yet, "they seemed like only a few days to him because of his love for her" (Genesis 29:20). This is not the familiar, cozy kind of love that we extol today in Western society, but the kind of deep longing and desire that has a man pine so deeply for a woman that it transports him above time and space.

If desire is the most important ingredient in any relationship – and I am convinced that it is – then sex becomes the most important barometer by which the success of a relationship can be measured.

Sex almost always wears off in marriage. Every study shows its frequency declines substantially as the years drag on.[5] We make peace with that decline through subterfuge and deceit. We start talking about being best friends rather than lovers and other euphemisms that are meant to compensate for the loss of passion. But there is no denying what is actually taking place. Two people's yearning for one another is wearing off.

So how can it be sustained? This is the billion-dollar question. Can two people who start off deeply in love sustain the same level of mutual intoxication, and even have it grow, as they spend more and more years together? If it can't be done then we have to question the very institution of marriage itself, as millions are now doing, with a recent study by Pew Research showing that 40 percent of all Americans now believe that marriage is obsolete.[6]

I reject such pessimism utterly and believe not only that marriage is the single most beautiful relationship in all human existence, but that passion in marriage can actually grow with time. I have invested a significant portion of my life to fathoming how and sharing it with the public.

In the course of this book we will examine the state of the union. We will look at the ways that marriages are suffering, and I will prove to you that the problem stems from basing our marriages on love instead of lust. We will come to understand why many married women are sexually stifled, and why so many men are looking outside their marriages – whether through affairs or through Internet porn – to satisfy their sexual needs. We'll explore the nature of lust and come to understand what it really is and what fuels it. We'll look at the reasons why we as a society negate the value of lust and misunderstand its value. We'll examine biblical marriages and I'll show you how the Hebrew Bible considers lust within a marriage necessary and even holy. I'm going to reveal to you the three principles of lust and show how each of these principles can be brought into a relationship so as to maintain long-term covetousness. We'll discover how lust can be applied to other realms beyond the physical, and even used as a marketing tool! I will show you how lust is based on polarity, and we'll talk about how to reintroduce that concept into our relationships and our society. We'll discuss the ultimate purpose of lust and look at the incredible restorative spiritual experience that our marital relationships can become. And finally we'll establish a working model for how a marriage can practically integrate the dimensions of love and lust to make our marriages and our lives both resilient and joyful.

My core concept – that *lust and not love is the true foundation of marriage* – is hard for many people to accept. I'm asking you to make a serious paradigm shift in the way you understand relationships, and you're going to have to undo some programing in order to internalize this. So read the book as we develop the theme, talk it over with your spouse, let your subconscious mull it over. And then I'm convinced you're going to see an incredible revitalization in your relationship, and even in your life.

PART I

Unavailability: The Loss of Lust in Our Lives

Chapter I

Love Won't Keep Us Together

Love: The Downfall of the American Marriage

Marriage has never been challenged as much as it is today. In 1960, 72 percent of the American population was married; in 2010 that number had fallen to 51 percent.[7] Most Americans actually do marry in the course of their lifetimes – the number of people over age thirty-five who have never married has remained fairly consistent over recent decades at just 7 percent of men and women in 1970, and 10 percent of women and 13 percent of men in 2008.[8] That means that around 90 percent of Americans still tie the knot at some point in their lives. But close to half of those marriages end in divorce after a median duration of eight years.[9]

I've long maintained that any society that has a 50 percent divorce rate arguably doesn't have the right to call itself civilized. Don't you think it's kind of uncivilized living when one out of every two American couples who professed undying love suddenly become indifferent, or else hate each other's guts enough to fund lawyers to destroy one another (with children often suffering in the mix)?

Significantly, people are waiting longer and longer to take

the plunge. The median age for an American woman getting married for the first time is now 26.5 and for a man 28.7; in 1960 the median age for a blushing first-time bride was 20 and a groom 23.[10]

One of every three American men over the age of 35 is single; two in five women in the same category are.[11] This doesn't mean people aren't pairing up. They are, but increasingly without the formality of marriage. This has serious consequences for children. Since 2008, some 41 percent of all births in the United States have been to unmarried mothers.[12] Among women under age 30, most babies (53 percent) are now born out of wedlock.[13]

And this is not just an American problem – whole regions, like Scandinavia, have marriage rates around two-thirds those in the US.[14] (A 2005 article quoted a Norwegian woman who opined, "The idea of the holiness of the marriage has disappeared because there are so many broken marriages."[15]) And many South American countries hover at half the US marriage rate.[16]

Heterosexual marriage has fallen so much that we rarely even discuss it. We talk day and night about gay marriage. The only men who still want to get married in America are gay! As to the straight guys, conversations with their girl-friends might go something like this: the girl turns to the guy and says, "Look, I don't know how to approach this subject comfortably, but now that we've been dating for about half a millennium, is there any chance that maybe you think we ought to tie the knot and get ma–" and as soon as that first syllable comes out of her mouth he's already broken out in hives and is hyperventilating.

Look at the language we use: the *institution* of marriage.

Do you want to be institutionalized? Marriage is "settling down." Well, that sounds like an inviting prospect, huh? Before I was "living it up," but now I'm going to "settle down" and get into the drudgery and monotony and predictability of a committed relationship.

People now cordon off the better part of their twenties in order to date recreationally, just to push off that giant commitment, so that they can have some time that they *enjoy* in their life before they *settle down*. Young people seem to be saying, "I don't really want to do this (get married)," because married life looks like such a drag. Committed relationships appear to require a lot of work. They don't proceed naturally. They lack joy. And people feel they work during the day at their jobs; they don't want to come home to more work. People can barely summon the energy to find the TV remote, let alone swing from the chandeliers.

This generation craves its adrenaline fix; we love excitement. We don't want to be reduced to a life where the most action we can expect is movie night once a week on Saturday. If the best we can hope for in married life is a weekly Hollywood-induced fantasy that allows us to escape the grind of daily life, then why bother?

So how did we get to this state? What happened to marriage? You'll see many different studies attributing the problem to many different things. I want to get to THE reason that marriage is floundering.

What we've heard until now is that marriage is dead for the following reasons: Women are liberated, financially independent, so they are no longer willing to settle for marriage with a man who is beneath their standards. Women are no longer prepared to remain in a marriage that is not happy because they have the financial wherewithal to leave an unhappy marriage and pay the bills on their own. The dependence that was once associated with marriage is no more.

That explains nothing.

That doesn't explain the breakdown of love in the relationship. That just explains why a miserable wife *no longer has to remain* in a miserable marriage, but it doesn't explain *why she's miserable* in the first place.

We've heard other explanations: the death of tradition, the death of religion. Marriage is still seen by many as a more traditional, more religious institution. But that also explains nothing, because all the studies show that even among secular people, getting married is actually a very important priority.

Overwhelmingly, people still look forward to marriage. And this even among young people in college whose romantic relationships are so informal that they are described as "hooking up." This is a fascinating phenomenon, the hookup culture on the American campus. For me, hooking up is what a U-Haul does with a station wagon. I don't know how this now denotes the closest interaction between a man and a woman. But even in that hookup culture, where male-female relationships are on such a low level of commitment and formality, marriage is still something that people aspire to.

Since 1976, teenaged respondents to the University of Michigan's annual Institute for Social Research survey "Monitoring the Future" have been surprisingly consistent in their positive attitude toward marriage. In 2012, 84.5 percent of the girls and 77 percent of the boys indicated they expect to marry in their lifetime.[17] This was actually an increase over the corresponding figures in 1976–1980, when 82 percent of girls and 73 percent of boys said the same.[18] Similar results have been observed in the University of North Carolina's Carolina Population Center National Longitudinal Study of Adolescent Health, in which 83 percent of respondents agreed in 2008 interviews that it is "important" or "very important" to marry.[19]

The greatest proof that people still aspire to marriage despite all these arguments that marriage is no longer in vogue is that Hollywood – which captures the zeitgeist of the American culture – holds up marriage as the ideal. Nearly every romantic comedy ends with a wedding. Seeing the couple marry at the end leaves you with a warm, fuzzy feeling. It's the movie showing that the relationship *worked*; it led all the way to marriage.

> What ruined the American marriage is something called *love*. Modern marriage is standing on a faulty foundation. Simply stated: love is not enough to keep a man and a woman under the same roof for the duration of their lives.

How can we explain that people still want marriage despite its high failure rate? If people want to get married and consider it the ideal, why isn't it working?

I believe that what has most destroyed the institution of marriage is what we would least expect. Namely, what ruined the American marriage is something called *love*. Modern marriage is standing on a faulty foundation. Simply stated: love is not enough to keep a man and a woman under the same roof for the duration of their lives.

I know this is a strange statement, because in our culture, we have glorified love so much that we're convinced that it's the world's strongest bond, and as such, it should be a strong enough adhesive to bond a couple in happily wedded bliss for decades.

But I can give you one example that shows in a nutshell that there's something much stronger than love: people cheat, even though they love their spouses.

A Force Much Stronger Than Love

I counsel many couples who are trying to regain trust in their marriages after one of the spouses has been unfaithful. On my TV show *Shalom in the Home*, broadcast on TLC, we tried to have a different theme every single week, but the dominant theme, unfortunately, was infidelity.

The primary reason why women were thought to cheat in marriage was neglect, although this is a notion that is now being seriously challenged by extensive research. But by and large, whether for reasons of biology or propriety, women generally refrain from cheating on a husband they are in love with and who focuses on them romantically. Women, seemingly, are mostly satisfied to be monogamous in a marriage where they are doted on, where their romantic and sexual needs are addressed and they feel special.

With men, that's not the case.

When I sit with couples after the man has cheated on his wife, I ask a simple question: Why did you do it? Why did you betray the woman who is the mother of your children? Why did you violate the holy covenant of marriage? Nine times out of ten the husband turns to his wife and says, "I love you. I didn't love her." It's almost a cliché; the husband who's broken his wife's heart by having a one-night stand or an affair protests that he loves his wife; the other woman meant nothing to him, he'll say. In fact, 56 percent of men who cheat (and 34 percent of unfaithful wives, by the way) say their marriages are "happy" or "very happy."[20] So then why did he do it? He may not have loved the other woman ... but he *lusted* after her. He loved his wife but he desired his mistress.

So we see here that *lust is stronger than love*. A man can love his wife, he can be happy or even "very happy" in his marriage, and yet he can still be susceptible to sexual infidelity. Why? Because the power and the pull of lust is an overwhelming force that makes people forget everything in the wake of its magnetic tide. A man in the throes of lust for another woman will betray the mother of his kids, forget the holy covenant of marriage that he has pledged her, lose all sense of his moral obligations in a white hot instant, because love doesn't stand a chance when it comes to overpowering lust.

> The power and the pull of lust is an overwhelming force that makes people forget everything in the wake of its magnetic tide.

We're talking about a force so potent that people literally feel unable to resist it, even when the consequences may be utterly disastrous. How many state secrets have been given over in the arms of a seductive spy? How many powerful men have been brought down after succumbing to a sexual whim? How many women have lost their positions and fallen from their pedestals on the altar of lust? People in the grips of lust are unable to control themselves and can think of nothing else; men will risk a presidency; women report being unable to take care of their children and will make spectacles of themselves.

Great writers have always known which is the most powerful force in the universe. Try to name a woman in literature, with the exception of Lady Macbeth, who is famous for being in love with her husband. All the famous characters are adulteresses. The world's great literature is never about love. *Anna*

Karenina, Madame Bovary, Tess, Lady Chatterley's Lover are all novels about the power of lust.

Why would we want to leave a force this strong just for adulterers? I maintain that we can harness this force for our marriages and completely revolutionize them.

The Core Issue

Marriage is in such a sad state today because we haven't been bringing the power of lust into it. *The modern American marriage is built on love when it should be built on lust.*

> Marriage is in such a sad state today because we haven't been bringing the power of lust into it. *The modern American marriage is built on love when it should be built on lust.*

A library of books – tens of thousands – have been written about how to have a better marriage. More books on this subject have been published in the last fifty years or so than in the previous five thousand years of recorded history. With all that glut of information we are more clueless than ever.

Why? Because these books are not dealing with the foundation. They're all about how to increase love, how to increase friendship, how to have a better partnership. None of them discuss how the very foundation of the relationship has to change away from love and back to lust.

Spouses should certainly love each other, and they should certainly be friends with each other. You have to be able to discuss things in a congenial atmosphere and feel the warmth of constant companionship. Husband and wife should be comfortable together and able to work as a team in the day-to-day management of their lives. But that's only one dimension of the relationship. And it's not the most critical dimension. The unbalanced degree to which friendship and companionability has been elevated in the American marriage is stripping marriage of its passion and verve. It's creating relationships that are stultified, stifling, and lacking the core element that brings life to the marriage.

The most important ingredient in a happy marriage is desire. A man and a woman marry because they want each other. They desire to be together. Once that desire is lost, once their mutual lust wanes, once their curiosity for one another dissipates, they slowly drift apart.

> The most important ingredient in a happy marriage is desire. A man and a woman marry because they want each other.

In neutralizing the natural sexual tension that exists between man and woman in favor of morphing into one unisex homogenous entity, men and women snuff out the fire of their relationships. They choose a road of constancy and predictability, and they get marriages held together by the tepid glue of friendship as opposed to the fiery and scorching fusion of lust. No wonder that the leading cause of divorce today is falling out of love rather than argumentativeness. No wonder that monogamy has become synonymous with monotony.

Women feel old before their time. Men too feel deadened. Today's marriages lack vitality. They have been stripped of the electric current that should pulse between a man and a woman.

Ours is a generation that eschews tension and seeks inner beatitude. This accounts for the success of books like Eckhart Tolle's *A New Earth*, a resurgence in mind/body practices such as yoga and transcendental meditation, and the increase in the number of people who use medically prescribed anti-anxiety medication. But as my friend Dr. Mehmet Oz has said to me, "We need to become comfortable being uncomfortable."

We have paid a price for this deadening of the inner spirit as we have sought to silence our anxiety and to make all of our inner parts cohere. In an effort to squelch our feelings of inner turmoil, we have also shut down disquiet's brother: sexual tension.

The loss of libido in our time is largely attributable to the purging of inner erotic tension in pursuit of a deadening bliss. This is not only true in a practical sense, as in the case of a couple who climb into bed at night and rather than feel the electricity of erotic attraction instead pop on the television and slip into a Hollywood-induced coma. It is especially true in a philosophical sense. For sexuality is the friction of the masculine and the feminine, of the body's yearning to break free of its bounds and merge with another spirit. Tension and peace must coexist to sustain happy, long-term relationships.

Did it ever strike us that sexual tension is a spur to human growth? The ancient Greeks identified Eros as the overall desire to know.[21] The sexual urge is the life force itself. Once purged of tension, we become less animated and less alive.

Yet much about modern relationships is geared toward a purging of that tension. We drink to pacify ourselves, take drugs to deaden ourselves, pop Prozac and Zoloft in the aim of making ourselves feel calm and even and tension-free.

In lectures throughout the world, I ask singles to choose what is more important in a relationship: compatibility or attraction. Ninety percent choose the former over the latter, thereby selecting the easy integration of sameness and resolution over the charged friction of sexual polarity – a death sentence for a relationship. Men and women define a soul mate as someone with whom they have the most in common. They marry a doppelganger, create harmony, and work on the intimate orchestration of separate halves.

This does not mean you shouldn't have things in common with your mate. It's about recognizing that the glue that brings you together and keeps you together is not the cozy sameness you share. The genders are naturally opposite. I guarantee you that no matter how much a husband and wife have in common, they are intrinsically polar opposites. The differences are already there; the problem is in the lack of emphasis on those differences. When a couple focus only on their homogenous sameness, their life can become lackluster very quickly.

It's understandable (though not inevitable, as we are going to see) when this happens to a couple who have been together for a while. But in my role as a couples counselor and an author of many books on relationships, I am increasingly confronted with a far more upsetting and tragic trend. Increasingly I am seeing the hollow-eyed gaze, the limp and exhausted expressions, the utter lack of passion in women who are still in their twenties, who are just beginning their lives. Women with the bloom of girlhood still in their cheeks, but not in their hearts. Women who have been married for only a year or two and already feel used-up and cast aside. The idea of living the rest of their lives – sixty or seventy years – as a dried-up husk of a woman is too much to bear, and they begin looking for an escape hatch. Or they begin to shut down completely. The marriage becomes a slog while there's still wedding cake in the freezer.

Something has happened to these women, probably

without their even realizing it. They used to be women whose sexuality was a raging fire; they've become wives who have boring sex on their anniversary for ten disappointing minutes. But that's just what being an adult is, they think. They have vague, distant memories of the passions that used to course through them – just enough of a memory to serve as a constant, aching reminder of how rich and vibrant their lives used to be, how suffused with longing and excitement. Love is still there, but the passion is long gone.

As I sit with them, I know exactly what's happening, even if they are afraid to admit it or don't know it themselves. The fire has gone out in them. They exist but are not alive. They enthusiastically tackle the day – they have no choice but to honor their responsibilities – but they fear deep down that every day will be the same dull, uneventful grind. They have little to look forward to, so they fill their lives with endless frenetic activity. There is taking the kids to school and then to after-school activities, play dates, and birthday parties. After a while they are no longer women but just wives, no longer females but just mothers. Their own search for passion and excitement has been entirely subsumed under the rubric of being a mom and they live vicariously through their children.

Men, too, are suffering the effects of the listless, lustless marriage. They are providers and fathers. Like good modern men, they try to participate in childcare and domestic work. Somehow no matter what they do, it is never enough, and they have the feeling their wives are always looking at them with an air of disappointment.

To distract themselves from the existential meaninglessness, they may become online gaming fanatics, spending all their free time staring at a glowing screen. Many men turn into couch potatoes, addicted to television and all forms of spectator sports, looking in from the outside at lives that seem to have the excitement their own lives so desperately lack. When they do make love to their wives, they may try to bring some thrills into a dulled relationship by fantasizing about other women. Unfortunately they may escape the torpor of their lives in more destructive ways, resorting to pornography or even seeking sexual fulfillment with other women outside the marriage.

The strange thing is, on the surface, in many of these marriages nothing is wrong. No one is cheating. They love each other. There is no shortage of mutual respect – women, after years of struggle, are finding their opportunities in the workplace equal, and sometimes superior, to those of men. And men have no problem with it. They support their wives. They are good parents together. They are best friends. Why can't they make the passion last?

It breaks my heart to hear it, but these couples, in their desperation, often blame the institution of marriage. They were told by society that it was a bond of love and passion, but it has turned out to be just another kind of work. There's the mortgage to deal with, there are crying kids, there are a million little things around the house that need to be repaired. But they're stuck. They're married. This is their lot. They stop fighting the dullness of life and the fire inside them goes out.

Some people can continue coasting along like this for many years. But there is no masking the sense of dullness that has entered their lives. They have given up on having a true, passionate lover and have instead settled for a partner, loving and respectful to be sure, but a businesslike partner nonetheless.

Worse, they sometimes blame love itself. Perhaps love, they say, the most powerful and mystical experience there is, is simply not strong enough to carry us through life. Perhaps love is just a trick played on us by evolution to get us to procreate. Perhaps passion is destined to fade. And once it has, love casts us aside.

Such an idea strikes despair into the heart. We have a primal, fundamental need for connection. As God said in Genesis 2:18, "It is not good for man to be alone." If love is not enough to break us out of our isolation and join us together with another soul, what is? Perhaps it's hopeless.

I spend a lot of time counseling people to fight against this seductive, existentially bleak argument. Love is certainly not hopeless.

At the same time, it's not really love that brings two people together. We don't long to do someone's dishes. Does a man bring a woman flowers to convince her to let him change the oil in her car? Does a woman watch her figure and wear makeup so that she can be granted the irresistible opportunity to iron a man's shirt?

Of course not. Our supposedly "higher" impulses do not attract us to our mates. We do not come together because we are longing to care for someone's soul and spirit through long, deep, thoughtful conversations, however sublime this may be. We do not fall in love because we see our beloved's spiritual essence, or because we discover how love makes us better people. (That comes later.) If we are honest with ourselves, what brings us together is a raw, almost crazed longing to connect with another human being in the most passionate manner possible. We are drawn to the object of our desire, whom we long to know in the deepest, most carnal way.

Yet the American libido is on life support.

A sexual famine is gripping America, with one out of three long-term marriages being entirely platonic[22] and the remaining couples having sex about once a week for seven to ten minutes at a time.[23] Our libidos are in the doldrums. Man has forgotten how to make love to a woman. And people have forgotten how the dynamics between men and women are supposed to work.

> It's not really love that brings two people together. We don't long to do someone's dishes. Does a man bring a woman flowers to convince her to let him change the oil in her car? Does a woman watch her figure and wear makeup so that she can be granted the irresistible opportunity to iron a man's shirt?

To be sure, both friendship and lust are necessary. The complete marriage is where husband and wife are both lovers and best friends. But today we are mostly, and sometimes only, the latter. Friendship, however, is not the nuclear bond that marriage requires in order not just to survive but to flourish. I wrote my book *The Kosher Sutra* in order to establish the eight principles of eroticism so that married couples can bring lust back into their relationships. But modern marriages for the most part are missing this crucial element. Modern men and women don't have a deep understanding of the erotic mind. Not only is this sad, but it also explains, in my opinion, the reason that marriage is dying as an institution. It seems so boring and routine.

The antidote to this lackluster existence is true lust, passion, vitality.

That's what we're going to discover in this book.

Chapter 2

The Sexually Extinguished Wife

A Woman's Primary Need

"The great question that has never been answered, and which I have not yet been able to answer, despite my thirty years of research into the feminine soul, is 'What does a woman want?'" Sigmund Freud wrote in a letter to Marie Bonaparte in 1925.[24] Even after three decades of being privy to women's most intimate thoughts, the world's most famous psychiatrist still did not know what a woman wanted. Most husbands say the same.

But right now, right here, included in the price of this book, we're going to answer it. As a man deeply in touch with his feminine side, I'm going to offer insight (I hope my wife doesn't read this and start laughing). Ready for it, guys? Ready to make history? Here's the answer: A woman wants to be intensely desired. To be lusted after. To be *chosen.*

In marriage, women are not looking just for love; rather, they are primarily looking for lust. A woman wants to be wanted, desires to be desired. A woman does not go into marriage principally to be loved; she goes into marriage to be lusted after, to feel that there's a man who has a magnetic attraction for her. It's an easy point to prove. If a woman wanted primarily to be loved, why would she ever leave the comfort of the parental home? No one's ever going to love her more than her parents. Her parents are never going to divorce her. Her parents aren't going to cheat on her. We never hear of Mrs. Jones going secretly to the next door neighbor's kid in the middle of the night and saying, "Heather, you're the daughter I really wanted. My own daughter doesn't understand me. One day I'll be able to celebrate my parental love for you in public. But for now, here's a secret dress I bought for you." Cheating on our children is a preposterous idea. A young woman's parents are going to love her unconditionally. She doesn't have to dress up for them; she doesn't have to impress them. They love her no matter what she does. If you want to be loved, you stay at home.

Freud said he did not know what a woman wanted. Most husbands say the same. Ready for it, guys? The answer is *to be chosen*. To be intensely desired. To be lusted after. A woman's primary need is to be desired.

So why is it that by the time she's a teenager her parents have to *threaten* her to be at home? Why does she trade in the unconditional love of her parents for the very conditional love of a man? It's because her parents have a genetic gun to their heads making them love her. They love her because they have no choice, and that's why their love can't make her feel special. When her parents tell her she's the prettiest girl in her class she just rolls her eyes. She doesn't believe them. They're not objective. They're just saying that because they're her parents. But when a man says that to a woman it must mean that she's special, she's unique. Her parents can give her love but they can't give her what she *really* wants, which is to be *chosen*.

To be chosen is to be made to feel special. You're chosen because you're unique. You stand out. You're intrinsically special. Created in the image of God, you reflect His uniqueness. He is the one and only and there is someone who makes you feel like you are too. That's why the Jewish people are referred to not as God's beloved people, or smart people, but "chosen" people. It implies that they are selected for a mission of spreading the Ten Commandments and teaching morality to all nations, which gives them a unique distinction in informing all of God's children of His love for them.

Chosenness is the one gift that parents cannot give their children, and that's why women are willing to leave the unconditional love in their households of origin and gravitate toward marriage. When a man marries a woman, he is announcing to the entire community, in front of God and all his friends, that he is choosing this one woman. She's the one who is the most special to him. She's the one he wants.

How about the old stereotype that women want to be supported and taken care of – that all they want is a rich guy who will shower them with diamonds? I have counseled women like this, who married rich men who love them and take care of them, but don't focus on them romantically. Happiness for them is a challenge. They will remain in their marriages and refrain from having affairs in order not to risk their stability, but they are bereft because they lack the one thing they want most: to be desired.

In the Hebrew language there is a specific word for "husband" (*baal*), but no specific word for "wife." The word used to identify "wife" (*ishah*) is exactly the same as the word for "woman." A "wife" is in essence a "woman." She never fully becomes a wife. A woman is always a woman, no matter who she is and what role she plays in life. She retains an insatiable nature that can never be fully controlled. She can never be fully possessed, even in marriage, which, ironically, is a good thing. It means that no husband can ever take his wife for granted. Even after you marry her she never fully becomes your wife. She remains a woman who can only be won over not by the commitment of the marital institution but through the daily solicitation of emotional devotion and affection. A woman, being a woman, responds to the attention and love shown to her: she must be won over.

The point is best illustrated by the story of Bruriah, wife of the Hebrew sage Rabbi Meir. A daughter of the respected martyred sage Rabbi Hananiah ben Teradion, Bruriah is one of the few women singled out in the Talmud as being herself a sage. She was an intellectual, a righteous woman par excellence, and a paragon of faith who proved her mettle in soothing her husband's grief with complete acceptance of the will of the Almighty when their two sons suddenly died in tragic circumstances.[25]

A curious story referred to in the Talmud (*Avodah Zarah* 18b) only as "the Bruriah incident" has much to teach us about the traditional Jewish attitude toward women's sexuality. The eleventh-century canonic Jewish scholar Rashi comments on this cryptic reference as follows:

One time [Bruriah] mocked the Sages' saying "Women are suggestible" (*Kiddushin* 80b, *Shabbat* 33b). [Rabbi Meir] said to her: "In your lifetime, you will eventually affirm their words." He instructed one of his disciples to seduce her. [The student] urged her for many days, until she consented. When the matter became known to her she strangled herself, and Rabbi Meir fled out of disgrace.

Much ink has flowed over this unusual and heartrending account throughout the centuries. I'll give you my take on it. Bruriah heard her husband teaching his students the passage from the Talmud (*Kiddushin* 80b) that says "*Nashim da'atan kalot aleihen.*" It literally means that women are "lightheaded," but Rashi explains this to mean that they are sexually uninhibited and receptive, or in other words, as I have rendered the translation in its proper context, "suggestible," and indeed this appears to have been Rabbi Meir's intention. I imagine Rabbi Meir telling his students that husbands must not take for granted that their wives are permanently won over. *Rather, Rabbi Meir taught, women are profoundly romantically impressionable. A woman can't resist when a man focuses his starry-eyed attention on her, and therefore a husband must ensure that he himself is his wife's seducer.*

Bruriah took issue with the Talmud's assertion that women are readily seduced. *You're insulting women, she told her husband, by insinuating that we're not innately moral and some Don Juan can come along and sway us; it's not true. I am not primarily an emotional person, she said; I'm an intellectual like you. When I know something is wrong, it's an iron-clad conviction.*

"*B'chayecha*," in your lifetime, Rabbi Meir replied; *in your lifetime you will bear witness to the truth of this aphorism.*

Rabbi Meir set out to prove to his wife the Talmud's wisdom, tragically recruiting one of his students to seduce her to demonstrate the point. Bruriah resisted the young man, just as she had said she would. But the student was persistent.

We don't know whether the student had feelings for her or whether he acted only out of a sense of duty to his teacher. We also do not know precisely what it was that she consented to and whether she actually succumbed to the seduction. "When the matter became known to her," Rashi tells us, "she strangled herself." Did it become known to her that she had fallen for the seduction and proven Rabbi Meir's point? Or did it become known to her simply that her husband had set her up?

Either way, the resulting shock apparently caused her to take her own life. Why was she so irretrievably humiliated? One explanation is that she had compromised her moral core and couldn't live with herself. Another explanation is that she was afraid people would find out. I don't accept either of those answers, because this is the same Bruriah who buried two of her sons and saw her father burned alive for teaching Torah, yet she persevered in her faith. This was not a weak woman or one who was afraid to ride against the current.

I think the reason she was so crestfallen to the point of wanting to end her life was that her husband had been proven right: for all her pretensions to being someone who could overcome her emotions and passions and choose her own path, someone who was a master of her own destiny, guided only by the cold, hard facts of logical principles, she discovered that her passion in fact trumped her intellect. She became terrified of what she was capable of. It was her core femininity that she had to acknowledge. This was what Rabbi Meir had been saying to her that she had to accept, and that's why she took her life: she despised who she was.

Yet we do not share her low opinion of herself. Bruriah did not go down in Jewish history as a disgraced woman. On the contrary, she is honored until today by having children and schools named after her. My own daughters attended a high school in New Jersey named after her and my sister attended a seminary in Israel that also bears her name. We do not believe that her last act demonstrated she was a woman bereft of virtue. On the contrary, we continue to honor Bruriah not despite her last act but perhaps even because of it. There's no shame in being an emotional creature who cannot help but respond to the affections of a man. We endorse that vision of femininity. A woman is special because of her passions, her feelings, and her humanity. There's nothing to be ashamed of in being that kind of person.

But this, of course, does not excuse immoral action. Rather, the rabbis caution against an unmarried man and woman becoming too close and having to suppress the natural bonds of attraction that ensue. That's the real sin. Not that we are possessed of passionate natures that can burn out of control but rather that we refuse to acknowledge this truth and don't take necessary precautions to ensure that do not find ourselves in immoral situations. A famous Jewish saying goes like this: the difference between the clever person and the wise person is that the clever person can extricate him or herself from situations into which the wise person would never have gotten in the first place. When it comes to the possibility of infidelity and unfaithfulness, we must always seek to be wise rather than clever. We must place limits and safeguards on whom we interact with so that we do not find ourselves in compromising situations within which the natural bonds of attraction must be suppressed.

Bruriah was an unusually strong woman with an unimpeachable moral character. She prided herself on being a cerebral intellectual. She was not proud of her feminine nature.

But this incident shows that she could not repress her natural passions. Her response simply validates what Rabbi Meir said: women struggle not to respond to the life, the intensity, the intimacy, the passion, and the lust that are shown them. They are profoundly human. To the contrary, someone who doesn't respond to human emotion is someone we dismiss as robotic, inhuman, and cold. Ultimately emotions are superior to intelligence in that they are what connects us to other people. It's men who usually fear emotional intimacy and intensity. Wives have the ability to bring them out of that disconnection.

Ancient Hebrew scriptures support the belief that women are more sexual than men. A Jewish marriage contract actually spells out a man's conjugal obligations to his wife, and not vice versa. Western sources historically tended to concur with this view, considering women to be less rational than men and thus more susceptible to passion.[26] Christian religious thought recognized this tendency but saw it as uncontrolled and threatening; the Dominican monk and inquisitor Heinrich Kramer wrote in his 1486 handbook *Malleus Maleficarum* that "all witchcraft comes from carnal lust, which is in women insatiable."[27] By the eighteenth century, an important shift in thinking had occurred: women were still considered highly impressionable in sensual matters, but the emphasis was now on protecting their inherently prim nature from such influences. Church of England clergyman Josiah Woodward expressed the view that women, with their "Weak and Tender Minds," should not attend the theater lest they be swayed by the sexual immorality and wantonness displayed there.[28] By the nineteenth-century Victorian era, the stereotype of "female passionlessness"[29] had become well established. Any diversion from what was seen as proper behavior was labeled pathological. Women were diagnosed as nymphomaniacs for behavior such as "committing adultery, flirting, being divorced, or feeling more passionate than their husbands."[30]

The twentieth century saw a revolution of attitude, as reported (and perhaps also influenced) by Alfred Kinsey's iconic reports on sexuality (*Sexual Behavior in the Human Male*, 1948, and *Sexual Behavior in the Human Female*, 1953). Women by and large are thought today to be at least as interested in sexuality as men. Indeed, new studies in the field of sexology show women to be much more sexually voracious than Western society has recently acknowledged.

Dr. Meredith Chivers, an assistant professor of psychology at Queen's University in Ontario, Canada, is at the forefront of laboratory studies that measure women's physiological sexual responses and compare them to self-reported feelings of arousal.[31] Her work shows an "omnivorous" female libido, with women responding sexually to images of every type of sexual activity there is – male, female, solo, animal (oh, my!), together, and alone.[32]

Daniel Bergner's book *What Do Women Want?* catalogs an array of evidence that women are far more preoccupied with sexual matters than the stereotypes would have us believe: the Nielsen ratings company reports a jump in female porn users from one in four to one in three, female fans make up the largest base of porn star James Deen's Twitter followers, vibrators are commonly seen on the shelves of such popular mainstream retailers as Walmart and CVS.[33] It turns out that women's libidos are very much alive, and wanting tending.

Suzanne was a married mother who struggled with trust and confidence issues ever since being abused by a relative when she was a girl. When Suzanne was about to turn 40 she started having something of a mid-life crisis. "Am I still beautiful?" she wondered. "Has my life amounted to any-thing? Do I even matter?" In Scott, a coworker at her office, she found a receptive audience when he began to compliment her and make her feel desirable, telling her how special she was. She discussed the budding attraction with a girlfriend, who warned her that unethical men like Scott prey on the insecurities of women like her.

Suzanne felt she didn't even know herself. Had the feelings of happiness in her marriage been an illusion? Was her new unhappiness real or was it a residual reaction to the abuse? Notwithstanding how much desire was shown her by her husband, did she have a fundamentally insecure nature that craved even more? Could she put the genie back in the bottle and go back to being who she was before, happy and content as a wife? Or had dark, deep longings been stirred within her that would not be quenched? In counseling with me she agreed that the best way forward was to discuss these emotions and confusion with her husband, who should be her principal confidant. I convinced her that her husband would respond lovingly to her doubts and I spoke to her husband to ensure that he would be a loving support. Her honesty drew her closer to her husband and their desire for one another became much stronger than it had been.

Women respond to desire. It's as predictable as the laws of gravity. This must be understood as an elemental fact: a woman goes into marriage to be desired. That's why if a woman is loved by her husband she can still be very, very lonely in a marriage if she feels he's not romantically focused on her. I know this, because I've counseled these women. "I know he loves me," the lonely wife will say, "but I still don't feel attractive or special or unique – I just don't." It is simply an intrinsic part of a woman's nature that in order to flourish, she needs to feel desirable and be desired. This is a woman's primary need in a relationship.

> Nicole, an attractive young woman who came to me for counseling, had been relentlessly pursued by men when she was single. They gravitated toward her good looks and she'd had bad experiences with men who treated her as a body instead of a human being. Disgusted with this behavior and frankly somewhat disdainful of men, she had chosen to marry Don, a rather uncharismatic but solid and stable man. Their early marriage had been satisfactory, if unexciting. Don was supportive, responsible, and gentlemanly – everything Nicole's earlier suitors had not been – but over time, Nicole had come to feel more and more neglected by Don's lack of romantic attention.
>
> "We're friendly with each other," she told me, "but I feel like I have a roommate instead of a husband. We hardly ever have sex, and I wonder whether he even wants me at all. In the beginning this was a refreshing change from being mauled by men who treated me like a sex toy, but now I'm not so sure anymore. I feel like an inanimate object, as if I've turned to wood. There is just no passion in my life. I feel dead."

Understanding this simple fact – that being desired is a woman's primary need in a marriage – would counteract the growing trend in female infidelity. Although in the 1920s 28 percent of American men and 24 percent of women committed adultery, by the 1980s researchers were finding that as many as 72 percent of men and 54 percent of women would be unfaithful to their spouses at some point during the marriage.[34] Recent research suggests that the gap between male and female levels of infidelity is closing.[35]

One woman, married to a rich man, told me that many of her friends speak of having an affair, responding to advances from men, because they don't feel desirable to their husbands. To the extent that they do not do anything about it, it's only because they make a simple calculation: Is this (experiencing lust) worth risking my marriage, my kids, my life as I know it? Those who remain faithful decide it's not worth the risk. Adultery is a terrible sin and absolutely ruinous in a relationship. It's a soul-destroying activity that ought never be contemplated. But consigning yourself to living without a lustful dimension to your life is not the answer. Rather, couples should seek to restore lust to their marriages. Sadly, too many women fill the emotional emptiness with materialism, choosing to shop and spend money. But the void remains.

I meet many married women who are in their twenties and thirties but lack that lustful dimension. Life is tiring them out. They're busy with jobs and kids. There is housework and bills. They become bitter and worn. Their lives lack an erotic spark that can give them added vitality. It's not that they don't love their lives. Certainly they don't regret having their kids. Rather, there is no balance. There is hard work during the day but no powerful electric current at night. They are desperate for a jolt to the system. As time goes on, and as their sex lives become dull or nonexistent, the spark starts going out of their lives completely. First they miss it. Later, they forget what it ever felt like.

Married at 28, Helen is not yet 35 with two young children. A paralegal who works hard during the day and is busy with the children at night, she always seems harried and exhausted. When you speak to her about politics or movies, her comments are almost always cynical. Everything always falls short. Nothing is ever good enough and very little inspires her. I hasten to add that she is not depressed. She always has energy and tackles her responsibilities with zest. She has just as much physical energy as she once had, but not nearly as much life. Eight years ago she was a magnified version of herself. I was therefore not terribly surprised when she confided in me that her husband had become a video game fanatic, spending two hours each night playing games against friends over the Internet. She started going to sleep alone without him.

The way she phrased it was this: "It's so sad to see Michael throw away his potential. I can't get through to him." Yes, that is tragic. She did not need to spell out the other tragedy. Here is a woman who married to feel loved and desirable. She found a man to be not just her legally wedded husband but her lover. A man who would touch her skin and make it tingle, who would slowly awaken the hidden fires within. All this would take away the daily pressures and responsibilities that weigh her down. Physical intimacy has the power to melt all the burdens and make us feel free again. But not Helen. All she had was burdens. She no longer even knew there was such a thing as uncontrollable desire and having a man take her to the mountaintop from whose summit all of life's problems look trivial.

Helen's experience is common for many women. So few woman feel lusted after that they become desperate. And that's why so many of them are now reading a book that has become a global publishing phenomenon.

The Fifty Shades of Grey Phenomenon

Newsweek did a cover story asking this simple question: Why is *Fifty Shades of Grey* so popular? For the past sixty years, feminism has said a woman needs a man as much as a fish needs a bicycle. That's a deliberately extreme portrayal of a simple feminist thought, but the basic idea is that men are superfluous. *We don't need men to pay our bills; we don't even need men to have babies.* (It's gotten to the point that *New York Times* columnist Maureen Dowd wrote a book called *Are Men Necessary?* and *Atlantic Monthly* senior editor Hannah Rosin wrote one called *The End of Men.*) So why do today's women – in droves – want to read a book about sexual submission to a man?

Women have worked hard to achieve parity with men and to achieve independence from them. They have even overtaken men in many areas. Sixty percent of all college degrees are awarded to women.[36] Many high school boys can't keep up with girls, even in subjects like mathematics and the sciences where the boys used to dominate.[37] Three out of the five past Secretaries of State were women.[38] And about two thirds of divorces are initiated by wives.[39] It's the women rejecting men much more than the opposite. Battle of the sexes? The men lost.

Yet now women are fantasizing about submission before men, obsessing over a book in which a young, liberated female college student signs an agreement to be totally submissive toward a billionaire businessman who wants to make her into his sex slave. And women are reading this in the tens of millions!

What gives?

Why are modern women reading *Fifty Shades of Grey?* Why would women read this at all?

The best answer they could come up with in *Newsweek* was that women today have so many responsibilities with work and home duties that they want to escape into a stress-relieving fantasy of a man making their decisions for them. "[I]s there something exhausting about the relentless responsibility of a contemporary woman's life," the article asked, "about the pressure of economic participation, about all that strength and independence and desire and going out into the world? It may be that, for some, the more theatrical fantasies of sexual surrender offer a release, a vacation, an escape from the dreariness and hard work of equality."[40]

The UK *Telegraph's* columnist had the same idea: "E.L. James's *Fifty Shades of Grey* enables women to take a holiday from their multi-tasking selves, and let someone else take charge for once," blared the article's teaser.[41]

In that case, why aren't harried wives reading a story about a woman who hires a housekeeper? Or a financial planner?

This is the degree to which we have lost any deep erotic understanding. Millions of women make a soft porn book go mainstream and our explanation is that it's because they want a story about a man who makes their decisions for them. Talk about desexualizing women.

Why are women really reading this book? What makes it exciting? What is enticing about the heroine giving up her freedom? Isn't that what women rebelled against?

The real story of Anastasia and Christian Grey is about a man who lusts after a woman so deeply that all his money and his stuff – his toys, his helicopters, his company, and material success – mean nothing to him. He just has to have *her*. This billionaire can have whatever he wants. But he wants this one woman. He wants her so badly that he obsesses over controlling her completely, making her submit, owning her, and taking complete possession of her. Nothing else matters; he doesn't want to ink any deals except her. She has to, *has to* sign on the dotted line agreeing to be his submissive or he'll wither away. In other words, *it is he who is her slave*, and not the reverse. He can't be without her. He must have her. He is utterly smitten.

> When a man wants a woman that deeply, she can't help but submit because that is what a woman wants more than anything else.

Fifty Shades of Grey is not ultimately about Anastasia's submission. Christian Grey is the one who is being dominated: he can't live without his submissive. When a man wants a woman that deeply, she can't help but submit because that is what a woman wants more than anything else. Being wildly desired touches the core of a woman's being.

So few women today have that experience that when they finally witness it – even in a book and even if it's happening to someone else – they go crazy. Women today simply aren't being lusted after. And that's why they're flocking to read this book, because they don't know what that feels like, and they know that it's what they most want.

The extreme sexual polarity in this book triggered an extreme reaction, especially for women, and even more especially for married women. The book touched a real nerve, because it got to the core of what women want to feel and what they're missing in their lives.

Lisa and Jeff came to me for counseling after Lisa had gotten way too close to another man. He said that Lisa was staying in touch with an old college flame and it made him feel emasculated. They were having major trust issues in the marriage. Jeff was devastated, and all the more so because he felt he had been a model husband. "I washed the dishes, I helped with the kids, I've done everything right," he said. "I feel so betrayed." Lisa claimed it was all innocent. "He's an old friend. Nothing more. You just have to get past it," she said. "Anyway nothing happened." But Jeff couldn't put it behind him. In fact, with her stonewalling he was getting angrier and angrier. By the third session we had together he was berating her, "I did all this for you. I was always there for you. I support the family. How could you do this to me?"

Lisa finally spoke, in a voice just above a whisper, and said, "Stop using my imaginary indiscretions to excuse our absence of romance. I don't want us to merely have a practical marriage, where you and I excel at taking care of the kids, being social with friends, and paying the bills. I want to feel like a woman. I want an exciting romantic life." Jeff was a considerate and devoted husband. But he had rarely expressed a pure desire for Lisa as the woman who made his heart skip a beat. Lisa wanted to be treated like a woman, plain and simple, stripped of all her other roles.

So many wives have husbands who rely on them for all the practical matters of life. And make no mistake, they're important. Like that famous song in *Fiddler on the Roof*, where Tevye asks his wife Golde if she loves him, and she responds that for twenty-five years she has kept house for him, washed his clothes, raised his kids, so that must mean she loves him. Love is absolutely found in practical matters; we dare not denigrate the importance of showing up for the daily work of running a household together. But it's still not enough.

Being lusted after cuts to the core of what a woman wants: to be desired fully, totally, and completely, in every possible way, especially sexually. And no woman should have this need catered to by some lowlife, desperate womanizer who seeks out lonely wives. They manipulate women into the false feeling that they want them when really they just want to use them. And it sometimes works, with tragic results, because it addresses a core feminine need that every husband must be aware of.

No matter how much a couple shares the practical realities of raising children and running a home, when the lights go out at night every woman wants her husband to turn to her with just that sort of fascinated desire. It's almost a cliché that a husband will say, "I do express sexual interest in my wife, but all she ever says is, 'Not tonight, I have a headache.'" But a man whose wife rebuffs him this way has not lit the fire that a wife seeks. He has not fanned the flames of her desire by showing her that he is erotically fascinated by her. In short, he has not truly lusted after her.

And women's fires are not lit in the absence of their husbands' lust. The phenomenon is amply illustrated in an anecdote related by Daniel Bergner in his book *What Do Women Want?* Psychology professor Dr. Marta Meana of the University of Nevada at Las Vegas told Bergner about a patient whose lover would tenderly seek approval for everything he did during sex, frequently asking, "Is this okay?" This was, unsurprisingly, "very unarousing" to his partner, who saw in this timid behavior no indication that her man was carried away by raw desire.[42] Such tepid treatment, over time, leads to a deadening of a woman's life force. Yes, women want sympathetic and caring lovers. But sometimes a woman just wants to be taken.

When men complain that their wives don't respond to their amorous advances, chances are they are approaching them as husbands rather than as admirers. They make the mistake of thinking that a wife wants primarily to be tenderly loved, when in fact she principally wants to be lusted after, not just loved and taken care of. The proof of this is that women who have supportive rich husbands who take care of their every need still have affairs and risk everything, when they are not being made to feel desirable by their husbands. This is what a woman thirsts to hear more than anything: "I desire you. I want to be physical with you. Your beauty is overwhelming to me. I cannot control myself around you. I find myself thinking about you constantly and I have to have you – I don't care what the consequences are. I don't care if we don't go to sleep tonight and we have to get the kids to school in the morning; there are no physical considerations that can suppress my desire for you." That's what women want and need to hear; that's what will melt a woman, because it taps into her core desire. A husband who approaches a woman without wooing her is not likely to get much of a response, because he hasn't addressed her core need.

Some men are troubled in this area by what's called the madonna/whore complex. The essence of this mindset is that some men can only see their wives as one or the other. The madonna can't be the whore. The woman who is the mother of your children is someone with whom you can't express your full sexuality; you can't tell her your deepest erotic fantasies – she might find you sick or think there's something wrong with you. Besides, the madonna is sanctified; she's above sexuality.

Interestingly, I usually see this attitude that it's objectifying and degrading to your wife to lust after her in men who prior to marriage were womanizers. They are reacting against previous actions and a lifestyle that led to their own self-loathing. They got tired of their own behavior, which they could not be proud of. When Shere Hite debated me at the Oxford Union she spoke about the phenomenon that men date the women to whom they're deeply attracted, but when it comes time to settle down, they marry women they are compatible with and not as attracted to. This obviously has real consequences for a healthy marriage: it creates a bifurcation where your wife is the madonna and you find a whore on the side (sometimes quite literally). This book is about removing that destructive bifurcation. The man who sees his wife and their relationship that way misses the deepest understanding of his wife. She has a side of her that wants to be treated as a woman with no other considerations at all. She is just waiting and pining and aching to be lusted after.

The Grand Extinguisher

The American wife is currently living largely through a sexual famine. Her erotic needs are scarcely addressed. Married to a husband who often dozes in front of the television and stumbles into bed after she is already asleep, her options are often pitiful. She can either choose to have an affair, which she is loath to do, or go quietly into the dark, empty, lonely night, which makes her old before her time.

How many married women look in the mirror and wonder

where their passion went? How many look back to their single years when they really felt alive, when they knew sexual yearning and erotic hunger? And how many question how their once-fiery libidos could have been so thoroughly extinguished? What happened to these women?

Marriage happened, that's what. Their husbands happened. And most husbands don't treat their wives with the passion and desire that Christian Grey expresses for Anastasia.

One of the most erroneous ideas about marriage is that husbands want sexually adventurous wives, wild seductresses with powerful libidos. The truth, however counterintuitive, is that the average man wants a safe and domesticated partner who shores up his fragile ego rather than a sexually voracious woman who will challenge him to take possession of her.

This subject touches a very raw nerve, and I know this is true because when I published an article on this subject,[43] it generated more than a thousand comments, many of them irately arguing respective sides in the great war of the sexes:

> Sounds like my ex-husband, except that once he had me where he wanted me, he decided not to bother with sex at all. I put on weight to discourage other men; eventually, I decided to lose weight for myself. He complained that now he found me attractive, which he didn't want to do; it made him think about me a lot.

> No matter what a man does it just seems that his wife eventually goes cold on him, so why bother? Life itself is challenging enough so why have more challenges at home.

> This is why there is so much need to control women's sexuality and reproduction. Our sex scares you.

And when children arrive, the husband becomes a second-class citizen in their own home. Children first, mother second...husband and lover may come much farther down the list.

I couldn't understand how and why I lost myself so profoundly. Where did my vibrant, sensual, cheerful, confident personality disappear to?

Yes, a woman turns off the sex AS SOON AS she is comfortable enough with the nice guy to know he's not going to immediately leave. That's all it takes.

All my ex-husband wanted was a wallet, housekeeper, and nanny.... It's amazing how people do not think to remain impressive to their partners.

Women tend to agree, and men tend to protest, but the fact is that a man complains that his wife is no longer interested in sex, all the while transforming her from a women into a maid, and from a mistress and lover into the housekeeper and nanny. Husbands, without even realizing it, sexually extinguish their women, all but guaranteeing that the men themselves will have to turn to porn, affairs, or fantasy for their own erotic thrills.

Make no mistake. They don't mean to do this and it happens subconsciously. But it's real nonetheless. Modern women are losing the sensuality of womanhood. They are relegated to the roles of caretaker, wage earner, housekeeper, and waitress. Wives are burdened with fatigue, boredom, and a listless inability to experience pleasure or satisfaction. This is the story of women without fire. Women who do not light up, who do not burn with passion, desire, or sensuality. It is the story of women who have been reduced to function and consumption. Women without soul.

A wife whose libido has been extinguished in this way is trapped in a double bind. If she acquiesces to becoming the functional but fundamentally uninteresting person her husband seems, subconsciously, to want her to be, she becomes unappealing to him and a shell of her true self. There is little room for her to express her authentic sensuality. There is little room for her to flourish, explore, or self-actualize. Why pursue beauty? Why pursue wit, insight, creativity, personal sensuality? Is she forced to choose between marriage and selfhood?

The individual psyche of the woman is particularly important to her expression of sensuality. To be desirable, to desire, she must be separate from her husband. She must have a sense of herself. She must know, at a visceral level, the presence and power of her beauty. Too much familiarity, too much functionality is antithetical to the decadence of pleasure. A woman wants to be wanted. She wants to be longed for, lusted after, and fantasized about.

Most husbands would vehemently protest that, to the contrary, they want their wives to be sultry and sexy. But regardless of what they say, what they often end up doing is turning their wives into haggard housekeepers.

Why would any sane man sexually extinguish his wife? Isn't a sexually alive wife exactly what he wants?

You might think so, but buried deep within the male psyche is the fear of not being able to fully possess his wife, not being able to control her natural attraction to other men, and not being able to satisfy a woman's sexual insatiability. This is made vividly clear in the response of men in Kenya to author Daniel Bergner when he asked them why they mutilate the genitals of girls in their tribe before they reach adulthood: "So our wives will be faithful," they told him "matter-of-factly."[44] Bergner likewise reports a conversation with Concordia University neuroscientist Jim Pfaus, who opines, "Why have we boxed in women's sexuality? Why do we keep women's desire relatively repressed? We men are afraid that if we open the box, open her control, we're opening ourselves to being cuckolded. We're afraid of what's inside."[45]

A husband's greatest fear is that as a man he will not be able to measure up, sometimes quite literally. This is especially true once men confront the sheer erotic power and multi-orgasmic nature of the female libido, which is so much more potent than a man's. By domesticating her, he robs her of her passion. He may now possess her without much effort because a part of her has died. Of course, in the process he all but guarantees that other women (including those found in the pages of porn) will excite him but his wife will not. By slowly extinguishing his wife's libido and making sex into a once-a-week encounter lasting seven minutes at a time (the national average[46]), he gains proprietary rights to her body but ensures that it will never be as exciting as Monday Night Football.

Moreover, men are often threatened by emotional connection because it's something that they are not taught to be good at, or are not socialized to value properly, or are just not wired to do the same way that women are. Marital intimacy is a potentially very intense doorway into emotional connection, especially as a relationship deepens over time, and many men fear that level of intimacy and subconsciously look to deaden the connection. Most men are uncomfortable with emotional nakedness. It makes them feel ... well, naked and vulnerable.

And all too often, in an effort to avoid that emotional intensity, they gradually fall into a pattern of shutting out their wives by drinking beer and watching football and leaving their "better halves" to occupy themselves with the kids and the laundry.

How tragic that the modern American male has little clue as to the consequences of his actions. Does he realize that by failing to compliment his wife he teaches her to think she is not special? Is he aware of the fact that by failing to buy her colorful clothing he makes her feel she is not worth the effort? Has no one told him that by glancing at other women in his wife's presence he makes her feel that she is not beautiful? And is there no friend of his who can tell him that when he has sex with his wife without at least twenty minutes of foreplay he ensures that her body will go through the motions but will never come alive with deep and intense emotions? Sex without foreplay is sex bereft of real sexual lust.

And why doesn't he see all these things himself? Because he cannot look past his own insecurity. He does not realize that he is uncomfortable being in a relationship that will really test his masculinity. He looks for challenges at work and on the sports field. But at home he looks for nirvana and bliss. A compliant wife will provide it. A seductress will not.

The sexually insatiable woman generates excitement for her husband, but excitement that is always accompanied by the pain and panic of incurable tension. His comfort zone is gone. He must now permanently pursue her and woo her. Forget having a roving eye for other women. He now has a roving eye for other men, seeing if his wife is interested in anyone but him. He fears he will have to compete against paramours even after he is married. Sexual tension may get a husband's engines revving, but it can also make him feel as though the floor is collapsing beneath him. He spends his days trying to impress his boss; does he have to spend the whole night trying to impress his wife as well? Give the man some peace! Did he not get married so he could enjoy a tranquil domestic existence? Why should he have to put on a show at home, too?

Given the possibility of awakening real desire in their wives, most men prefer to forego the passion and play it safe instead. So a typical man turns to the usual distractions – sports, television, alcohol – because being an armchair warrior grants him a feeling of unearned superiority, a sort of calm within the storm. He is a champion who has never had to compete.

If he sees his wife as a woman who could get another man in a heartbeat, not only does he have to worry about keeping her as his woman, but also about whether he is up to the job. And this he fears more than walking a tightrope over the Grand Canyon. To get out of feeling inept and inadequate, and more importantly, to stay in control, he subconsciously and systematically wipes the sexuality clean out of her.

Note that this is something of an illusion on his part. A woman's sexuality can be made to atrophy, but it never disappears completely. Because of the intensity of emotional connection that a woman feels in her intimate relationship, women have core erotic needs that are much stronger than a man's. Taking advantage of these needs, there are wretched womanizers, unconstrained by any dictate of morality, who can spot a vulnerable woman from outer space. So like the ember that can be fanned into a roaring flame, a woman's dormant sexuality is easy to awaken with erotic attention. A woman who is made to feel desirable once again will blossom with the full potency of her sensual nature.

But husbands are, to say the least, highly ambivalent about this state of affairs. As a man begins to recognize how his wife, like all women, is desirable to, and desirous of, other men, and that attraction increases commensurately with the degree to which she feels unappreciated or ignored, he will be shaken with feelings of inadequacy and anxiety.

Linda and Eric came to me with their marriage in a state of confusion. Eric was a faithful husband, a fine, upstanding guy who would never cheat on his wife. But he did have a habit of flirting with other women. He was funny and charismatic, and he enjoyed chatting with people and making them laugh. This drove Linda crazy with jealousy. She wondered if she was simply depressed.

In an effort to boost her self-esteem, Linda started working out with a personal fitness trainer. Brad was tall, buff, and handsome, and most of all he was totally focused on Linda. He would constantly compliment her, praising her efforts and telling her she looked fantastic. He would call her frequently to touch base about what she was eating ("Stay away from those carbs, Linda!"). If she went to a party, he would call her while she was there and ask her what the food was like and what choices she was making.

Brad took a wholehearted interest in Linda – unlike Eric, who made Linda feel loved but not desired. At first Eric encouraged Linda's workouts with Brad, seeing that Linda was losing weight and feeling good about herself. He said, "I'm not the jealous type; you're the one with that issue. This is fine with me."

In fact, when I asked once in a counseling session what Linda would most want from her marriage, she said she wished her husband would be more jealous.

She got her wish.

Eric began to notice that Linda was getting up early to go work out. She often talked about Brad and his opinions. "Brad says we should go here and not there for vacation," she would say. It was always Brad says this and Brad says that. For the first time in their marriage, Eric began to experience serious jealousy.

The dynamic of their marriage had shifted. Eric had always seen his wife as pursuing him. She was the one who was always jealous of him. But now he wished she were more jealous again! She no longer seemed to care that he was flirting with other women.

Linda was completely cured of her neurotic obsession with her husband's flirting by the attentions of another man, but at the expense of the intimacy of her marriage. Blooming with self-confidence and feeling desirable once again, she was fully awakened after years of subtle neglect by her husband. Eric, on the other hand, felt knocked off balance by his wife's renewed sensuality. He felt insecure and wished Linda would go back to being dependent, even lackluster.

Eric did not understand the nature of a woman. He did not understand that like Bruriah, the most virtuous of all women, a woman by her very nature is responsive to a man's desire for her, because it touches on her deepest need. What Eric also tragically did not understand is that a woman's craving for this type of attention is actually magnified through neglect. Would Linda have fallen for Brad when she was twenty-five years old? Unlikely. It was only because of years of feeling deadened by her husband's lack of focus on her that Linda was vulnerable to falling for the first sleazy guy who came along and treated her like a woman again.

Men are naturally competitive. They don't want to have to compete for a woman they've already won over. Sure, they want the erotic thrills that come from seduction and pursuit. But they also want to know, now that they're married, that they have a comfortable, safe haven to come back to. Men want to see their wives as already conquered terrain. They want to know that their wives are not attracted to strangers or attractive to strangers, at least not in a way that's dangerous or unsettling. Also, if they want to pursue their own erotic thrills by finding women outside of the marriage, they don't want to feel that their neglect will lead their wives to pursue other men in order to satisfy their own erotic needs.

Kathy came to me for counseling, distraught. Her husband Dave was a businessman who traveled a lot. He loved his wife and didn't want to embarrass her in their home city, but when he traveled, he really played the field. He was having sex with a lot of women on his trips. What he wanted from his wife was to look after the home front. If he had to worry about the home front, after all, he wouldn't be able to chase women.

I advised Kathy to turn her cell phone off every day after 5 p.m. "Your husband is assuming that you're safe, that he has nothing to worry about when it comes to your own fidelity," I explained to her. "You have to change the dynamics of your relationship." Well, Kathy took my advice and it made a huge difference. Her husband was immediately disturbed when he called and found her unavailable. "Where were you?" he asked her with great agitation when he finally reached her. "I was out with friends," she said. "Which friends?" he wanted to know. "Just friends, nothing important," she told him. "I'll see you when you get back. Are you having a good time?"

Dave became more and more concerned, deeply uncomfortable about her unavailability to him. He started canceling his business trips so he could be home with her more. As long as he thought she was "in the bag," he felt free to womanize and neglect her, but as soon as he started to see her as her own person with her own activities, he was racked with jealousy and doubt.

When Kathy made herself more mysterious and unavailable (we're going to discover more about that later), her husband stopped assuming that he could safely neglect her. He could only afford to chase other women when he felt there was ease and security in his home. When his wife, however, shifted the balance and created a lack of comfort on the home front, Dave was highly agitated. It is in the hopes of forestalling this kind of agitation that a man tries to relegate his wife to a totally desexualized realm. Much better, he thinks, to subtly and even subconsciously extinguish her sexuality.

What ensues is the boring domestication that most married couples suffer. Two people who live in the same house, share a life, share kids, have perfunctory sex, but never make love. Two people who are married but never generate true erotic friction.

Understanding the male aversion to this tension explains a powerful literary conundrum that has bedeviled critics for generations. Notice that many of the voracious, beautiful seductresses of classic literature end up dying a gruesome death. And it's always the male authors who wrote them into existence who end up killing them as well. As psychotherapist and cultural critic Dalma Heyn argues, from Tolstoy's Anna Karenina and Flaubert's Madame Bovary to Thomas

Hardy's Tess, these women excite their authors but make them so anxious that they have no other choice but to polish them off.[47] The unpalatable tension these women create in men is best addressed by their being dispatched. Tolstoy's biographer Henri Troyat makes a convincing case that Tolstoy actually fell in love with Anna as he created her.[48] But it was love accompanied by an unmitigated hate that could only be remedied by Anna's destruction at the hands of Vronsky's neglect. Anna cannot live happily ever after. Her destiny is to be sliced apart gruesomely on the train tracks.

These authors subjected their heroines to grisly horrors because their strong sexual inclinations and permissive natures made them objects of intense desire but of equal revulsion. Countless men would wish to have a woman like Anna Karenina as their wife. A woman of exquisite beauty with an unquenchable romantic spirit is the dream of every man. Or is she? A woman of such irrepressible and insatiable spirit can never be truly had and can slowly erode the already brittle male ego of even highly successful men, as Karenin discovered.

What every man wants is a contradiction: a woman who, on the one hand, makes his pulse quicken, but also one over whom he can exert ownership. He wants sexual excitement accompanied by domestic bliss. The two cannot easily coexist. The tension that arises in pursuit of this ideal is enough to drive a man mad. So he kills off the seductress in his wife. Some do it with threshing machines, as Hardy did with Tess; some do it with train tracks, as did Tolstoy with Anna; while others accomplish the same end by turning their wives into dishwashers and maids, avoiding them sexually and romantically until the wives lose all memory of their former sensuality,

and their passion and thus their very essence is slowly extinguished.

We forget that there is an essential difference between
men and women. From their earliest age men are judged, for
the most part, by their *doing* and women, mostly, by their *being*.
Men must earn the world's attention through achievement
and work. But women can do so simply by being attractive
and pretty. And yes, I know it takes a lot of work to be attractive, especially these days when women are given impossible
standards to uphold. Nevertheless, it is work that is channeled
into the passive state of being and looking attractive. After all
is said and done, a superficial world gravitates toward women,
however unfairly (and it is extremely unjust), based first on
their appearance.

Men must guile the world with their activity while women
can do the same in their passivity. Because of this, men live
with phenomenal inbred anxiety and substantial inner pain.
Women are attracted to "the man with a plan." Success is their
magnet. So men live with the permanent insecurity of not
being enough, of having to constantly achieve. Hence, they
loathe anything that increases that feeling of insatiability
and look for wives for whom they no longer feel they have
to compete. The seductress who is eyed by other men puts
husbands back into the arena of competition from which they
seek so strongly to escape. Is it any great mystery, then, that
most men avoid the subject by marrying a lover but slowly
transforming her into a best buddy?

Having understood that a woman's primary emotional
need is to be desired by her man, we can see that lacking that
electric connection is bound to have a very negative effect on
her. She will feel lonely. She may even feel angry.

From here there are endless ways for couples to enter a downward spiral: she does not feel desired and is perhaps subconsciously angry and rejected. She may be cutting to him, which emasculates him. He desires her less. She gets angrier, and also may become unhappy or even depressed. As a result she may put less effort into her appearance, causing his desire to decrease even more. Her anger then increases, his desire decreases some more, and unless this whole sorry cycle is stopped, the two of them will be headed for divorce court.

> When husbands avoid emotional and sexual connection with their wives, they should know that they are drying up the pleasure garden that the two of them could otherwise enjoy.

So it's very much in a couple's best interests to find instead an "upward spiral," where desire leads to more desire. It is widely acknowledged that "there appears to be some truth to the popular adage, Use it or lose it, when applied to sexual behavior."[49] Not only can abstinence actually suppress desire,[50] but women may even experience physical discomfort with the resumption of intimate activity after a dry spell.[51] In sum, as *Psychology Today* suggested, "the more you have, the more you want."[52]

Desire feeds desire. Positive intimate connection creates more positive intimate connection. Lack of desire, on the other hand, kills desire. When husbands veg out in front of the television, play online games, give their attention to other women (whether in real life or on a screen), and generally find a million and one ways to avoid emotional and sexual connection with their wives, they should know that they are extinguishing their wives' sexuality and drying up the pleasure garden that the two of them could otherwise enjoy.

And they should also know that withholding erotic attention in a subconscious attempt to extinguish their wives' sexuality may backfire in an immoral way if another man steps in to fill the void. A woman's primary need is to be desired by her man. If you're a husband, don't you want to be that man?

Chapter 3

What Men Are Looking For

Not Good for Man to Be Alone

Probably the biggest crisis men face in contemporary society is loneliness and a feeling of emotional isolation. It's not a new dilemma: this was the first pain experienced by the first man. Imagine, all alone in the Garden of Eden, with not a single other human being in existence in the world. Adam's loneliness wasn't just a lack of someone to talk to, however. He had God's presence, the ministering angels, a view the size of the whole world. Why would he be lonely? The source of Adam's loneliness was not a simple lack of company, but this: there was no one to make him feel significant. There was no one who needed him. There was no one who could appreciate, cherish, and lean on his unique gifts. In short, he felt redundant and nonessential. Loneliness results not from feeling there is no one to love us but rather from feeling there is no one who needs us.

The Midrash tells us that Adam was surrounded by angels with whom he was capable of conversing – in truth he had plenty of company. But angels are perfect creatures who have no requirements. They could never *need* Adam. He was not essential to their existence.

No angel ever approached Adam and said, "I'm having a

tough time at work and I'm feeling down. Let's go talk over a beer." There was no angel who experienced financial hardship and needed Adam for a loan. Most important, there was no vulnerable woman to make him feel necessary in her life, to comfort her; there was no woman who needed him to compliment her; there was no one who could confide in him. Adam felt that if he were hit by a bus (I realize that the Garden of Eden didn't have huge traffic problems), no one would miss him. And so God commented: "It is not good for the man to be alone. I will make a helper suitable for him" (Genesis 2:18).

> While a woman's primary need is to be desired, a man's primary desire is to be needed.

So God created woman – a flawed and imperfect person just like him – who had real needs. And the rest is history. Man has his "helper," and there is no need for him to be lonely anymore. Happily ever after, and all that.

But wait! Why are so many men still lonely, even when they do have wives? Why does a man who has a special woman still feel unessential? The deepest level of loneliness is the feeling of insignificance – to feel that you don't matter, and there is no one to even acknowledge that you feel that way – trapped and isolated in a cocoon of pain where no one can reach you. There is no one who can understand your pain. Loneliness results from feeling that if you fell off the face of the earth, no one would really notice. Your existence is not essential to any of the people around you.

Forget someone actually making you feel significant. Forget someone telling you, "You matter to me; I need you" – I'm talking about the feeling that there's no one even to acknowledge that you feel alone, that you're in agony. And this is the essence of why so many men feel sexually and emotionally distant from their wives: their wives – whether they are to blame or not – often don't make them feel like they matter or that they're important.

Sometimes this has tragic consequences.

Marty was married to Elizabeth for nearly twenty years when he lost his job. Marty's wife Elizabeth, a successful doctor, was supporting the entire family. Unable to find employment despite numerous interviews, Marty was suffering from plummeting self-esteem. Seeing her husband in crisis, Elizabeth tried to get him to talk. But Marty could not open up. Elizabeth began to discuss her feelings of helplessness with a male friend at the hospital who was also a doctor. They became closer and eventually had a full-blown sexual affair. Elizabeth justified it, feeling that her husband had shut her out.

When Marty found out, it was the final straw. He felt totally alone. It seemed to him that not a single person on earth cared about him. He deteriorated rapidly and, in a moment of total desperation, took his life. It was Elizabeth, whom I met a few years later at a conference, who told me this terrible story that could so easily have been avoided had Marty learned to share his pain and had Elizabeth learned how to reach him rather than connecting with another man in her husband's emotional absence.

I've been involved in the field of counseling relationships for some twenty-five years. I've noticed something interesting. Ten, fifteen, twenty years ago, I would sit with men and women who were in a relationship and the men felt at liberty to talk about how sexy other women were, right in front of their partners. They would do it humorously, facetiously, but they still did it. I remember sitting with a guy in Miami Beach – a happily married man, with a loving marriage and a wife who was very attached to him – but he would say right in front of his wife, "Look at all these women [on the beach] – I'm in pain, absolute pain, knowing I can't have them." His wife laughed. Apparently she was used to this, and it seemed to be something of a norm at the time. What I am noticing now, however, is that so many wives feel at complete liberty to talk in front of their husbands about sexy gorgeous hunks that they meet.

I was sitting with a couple in a social situation and the wife was telling her husband, right in front of me and everyone else, "You have no idea how incredibly cute this guy is that they just hired in my office." This woman is 35 and she was describing a guy in his late twenties. She was just going on and on about how amazingly hot this man was, and the husband kept casting glances at me as if to say, "Help!" Women feel at much greater liberty to discuss this today. So the tables are really turning. Is it payback? The glorification of youth? A growing amoral culture that shuns commitment? We always knew men wanted younger women. But now women are drawn to younger men. More so, however, it's an increasing phenomenon that men are simply seen as unnecessary (remember *Are Men Necessary?* and *The End of Men?*). With this as the prevailing social context, is it any wonder that men are experiencing an epidemic of existential loneliness?

Todd and Melissa came to speak to me separately, in turmoil after Melissa had gotten overly involved with her boss at work. Melissa's boss was a powerful man with a troubled marriage, and he used to confide in Melissa. The more he confided in her, the more she came to comfort him, and they began to spend hours talking about personal matters. Back at home, Melissa would bring up her boss a lot, which is one of the telltale signs of an emotional attachment that is forming.

There are four levels in addiction: use, abuse, dependency, and addiction. For months Melissa denied that she was growing through these various stages in her relationship with her boss. Meanwhile Todd was feeling very bad about himself. His wife was speaking to him less, speaking about the other guy more, and she would get all dressed up to go to work. Yet she denied anything was happening. In fact nothing physical ever happened between Melissa and her boss, but the emotional energy was depleted in her marriage. After many months of denying that anything was brewing, finally, after hours of conversation Melissa confessed to Todd that she had developed an unhealthy emotional attachment to her boss. Todd was so wounded at her dishonesty that he could not speak to Melissa for months.

When Melissa came to see me, she said that she couldn't understand why Todd could not forgive her. After all, she had not even technically been unfaithful! Then I spoke separately with Todd. "People lie about their affairs," I told him. "So she lied. It was wrong and highly immoral," I said, "and it's very painful. But she is now trying to take responsibility and you have to move beyond it." Todd looked at me with an expression of pure grief. "That's not it," he said forcefully. "It's not because she lied. That's not the reason why I can't open up to my wife. That's not the reason that I can't expose the contents of my heart to her. The reason is that she saw me in pain all these months, and not only did she not care but she didn't even notice. I was hurting for so many months, and she didn't even *see it or acknowledge my pain." Melissa's emotional infidelity had wounded Todd, but it was the fact that she didn't even see his pain, that she made no effort to understand him, that left him in a state of the most severe form of loneliness.*

There are three levels of loneliness. The first is aloneness, simply feeling detached from human company. It is easily remedied by hanging out with friends or joining a community. The second is classical loneliness, the feeling of not being needed, or having one's existence be rendered superfluous. That is remedied by being in an intimate relationship where someone else places you at the center of his or her existence. But the third kind of loneliness is the feeling that no one understands you. It's where you're alone in your pain and no one can reach you. This kind of loneliness is devastating, especially for a man, because it denies his core need. Feeling understood in your pain is part and parcel of feeling necessary. If no one tries to meet you in your pain (and men make it very difficult because they deny the pain, they don't open up), isn't that an a priori proof that you don't matter? If people don't even make an effort to find you in your pain, if they leave you alone in that pit to rot and die, doesn't that mean that you are insignificant, irrelevant, and nonessential?

This is why a man is devastated when his wife (whom he may even be neglecting and ignoring, by the way) turns to another man for her own needs. And it's not just the feeling of betrayal. Having a wife cheat on him devastates a man all the more because in some measure her infidelity strikes at the core of the male psyche.

Jessica and Ryan came to me with their relationship in tatters after Jessica had had a fairly short-lived affair. Over a period of several months, Jessica had developed an inappropriate relationship with another man, ultimately leading to her sleeping with him three times. When Ryan found out about his wife's affair, he was beside himself. Thoughts of her in another man's arms ruined his confidence and made him feel he had nothing to live for. In the course of counseling, Jessica, trying to comfort him, said, "You have to believe me, I never loved him. You're the one I love. It's just that this lust took over me – I was overpowered by this feeling."

Jessica was trying to comfort Ryan, but in fact her words made him feel so much worse. She was saying that no matter how much she loved him (and her genuine love was clear in her eyes), she had felt an explosive desire for this other man. In other words, this man brought out something in her that her husband had not. Ryan was devastated because he was hearing that his wife had experienced something with another man that she didn't experience with him.

A man wants to be the center of his wife's world just as she wants to be the center of his. He wants to be the one who does things to her she has never before experienced. He wants to be needed; he wants to be the one who brings out her fire. When he discovers that some other man brought out the womanhood in her, and she's changed as a result, he's deeply wounded. He's emasculated and despairing, because his primary need to feel needed has been violated.

Too often a man seeks affirmation of his being needed in other women's arms, or in workaholism or the pursuit of money, power, or fame. But a man who does not feel needed is simply crushed. Have you ever noticed that the stereotype of a retiree who has nothing to do but sit around and twiddle his thumbs until he languishes applies only to men?[53] Men also tend to suffer more from unemployment than do women.[54] A man, who is told all his life that he has to perform and produce and impress, feels vital when he feels *necessary*. Indeed, the word *vital* means both "full of life and vigor" and "of the utmost importance" (Merriam-Webster). They are two sides of the same coin, especially in the mind of a man. This is true in the workplace, and it is true in the bedroom as well.

Why Men Look Elsewhere

If a man needs above all else to be needed, and he has in his house a woman – his wife – who needs him, then why would he ever go outside the marriage? Why would he ever cheat? Almost everyone believes that a man who cheats on his wife does it primarily for sex. Men love sex. They crave and need variety. They can't control themselves. Mystery solved.

After the Tiger Woods cheating scandal broke, I was invited on CNN to discuss why he did it. The other male panelist on the show piped up, "Is this some kind of puzzle? The guy is rich. The guy is famous. He has unlimited access to all the beautiful women in the world he would want. And men love variety. They want a lot of women. So he slept with all those different women. There's your explanation. It's not much deeper than that."

It was my turn. "In that case, then, why did Tiger Woods cheat with the same woman over and over again? There was no variety here. Did you see the pictures of the more than ten women who had been identified as his girlfriends? They are all near exact copies of his wife. They are all blonde-haired, blue-eyed, Nordic-looking bombshells. But he already had that at home. So why did he go out and cheat with essentially the same woman? Where was the Asian woman, the brunette, the curvaceous plus-sized woman? No, they don't exist because he did not cheat in order to get variety. It's a shallow and incomplete explanation."

To be sure, men do crave variety. Women do too, but women tend to seek what I call vertical variety: that is, digging deeper into an existing relationship and finding something new (although, as I said earlier, that seems to be changing as women in our culture become more masculinized). Men are more prone to crave lateral variety, which can sometimes manifest in unwholesome ways such as affairs or pornography, because a new woman seems to satisfy the urge for lateral variety. (We'll talk more later about how men can find lateral variety within marriage.)

But as the painful Tiger Woods episode shows, there is much more to it than that when it comes to infidelity. In fact, men cheat not for sex but for validation.

Men don't cheat because they're liars and thieves. The vast majority of men who are unfaithful would never shoplift or steal a car. Rather, men cheat because, as Tiger Woods ultimately accepted in a press conference confession, they have a problem. They are broken on the inside – they feel insecure and unimportant – and think that having women desire them will compensate. That's why they need the variety. They get one woman to desire them, they consummate the attraction, and they still feel empty. So they try another, and another. Like a drug that ultimately doesn't take away the pain and must therefore be consumed in ever greater quantity, these men become womanizers in the hope that the endless parade of women will somehow make them feel whole.

It's the age-old lie that conquest, especially of a sexual nature, will bring personal validation. As Woods said, after all the money and fame he had earned, he thought that normal rules didn't apply to him. He was Caesar, which is another way of saying that even after all the fame and money he still was insatiable for more. All the accolades, all the fans, the beautiful wife, the adorable kids, still could not make him feel full. All the money still didn't make him feel rich. All the adulation still didn't make him feel worthy. He remained a black hole of endless consumption.

A man wants to feel powerful, important, on top of his game. He wants to know he's still got it. Somewhere along the line a cheating man's wife stopped making him feel special, stopped making him feel needed. Even making money does not make him feel special enough. On the contrary, the unending competition has made him even more insecure. Cars and other status symbols can no longer prop up his ego.

Men who cheat do not do so because they don't love their wives but because they hate themselves, not because their wives are not caring but because their perforated sense of self is immune to affection. Were their wives to shower them with all the love in the world, it would simply seep through the broken shards of their shattered egos. When first asked about the affair that would ultimately destroy his life, marriage, and career, John Edwards denied it by saying, "It's completely untrue, ridiculous. I've been in love with the same woman for 30-plus years and, as anybody who's been around us knows, she's an extraordinary human being, warm, loving, beautiful, sexy and as good a person as I have ever known. So the story's just false."[55] The form of his denial should have been a red flag. Men do not refrain from cheating because they have special wives.

Less so do men refrain from adultery because they are in love with their wives; incredibly, 56 percent of men who cheat rate their marriages as "happy" or "very happy."[56] Another study found that 80 percent of cheating men had no interest in leaving their wives.[57] Men find it easier than women to compartmentalize their commitments. Rather, when men refrain from affairs it's because they have a commitment to moral behavior and prefer the quiet pleasure of feeling noble, honorable, and committed to their wives over the illicit pleasure of sinful sex.

Like my fellow CNN panelist said: Men cheat. Get used to it. Case closed. But if there is no way to guarantee male faithfulness, why are we all scandalized when men do what Tiger Woods did? Further, a whole parade of powerful men – Eliot Spitzer, John Ensign, Mark Sanford, John Edwards, David Petraeus, Arnold Schwarzenegger, Dan Marino – are ruining themselves and their families with acts of infidelity. And we can't come up with any cause other than "powerful men have a sense of entitlement"?

What impedes any deep understanding of infidelity is the public's natural assumption that husbands have affairs for sex. In fact, the vast majority of husband's affairs have no physical component. They are cyber affairs that take place over the Internet. They are conducted over the phone and are never consummated. And even when they do get physical it is often very bad and unsatisfying sex, as Monica Lewinsky shared in the Starr Report and as a multitude of JFK's mistresses alleged as well.

In truth, men have affairs not for physical reasons but for emotional ones. Marriage counselor M. Gary Neuman, a fellow rabbi who is a friend, found that only 8 percent of cheating men cited sexual dissatisfaction as the main cause of their infidelity, while 48 percent of men said their primary reason for cheating was emotional dissatisfaction.[58] Furthermore, only 12 percent of the cheating men described the "other woman" as more physically attractive than their wives.[59] This puts the lie to the commonly held "wisdom" that men are unfaithful because they want sexual variety.

The truth is that men cheat not out of a sense of confidence but out of a state of brokenness. Not out of a sense of how desirable they are but out of a sense of what failures they are. And this is especially true of men like Tiger Woods and Bill Clinton who live in hypercompetitive environments where they realize that they are only special to the extent that they keep on winning. The public makes the mistake of assuming that powerful, successful men are the most confident, that elite sport stars like Tiger Woods are unflappable. Precisely the opposite is true. Everyone who seeks the spotlight, whether in sports, television, or politics, does so to compensate for some inner feeling of inadequacy. Their gnawing insecurity becomes the very engine of their success. Thus, they reason to themselves, if I become a rich businessman, a famous celebrity, or a powerful politician and get invited into high society, I'll be important.

Aristotle made clear more than two millennia ago, "Great men are always of a nature originally melancholy." Outwardly "successful" men are usually inwardly broken in some way, manifested in their reaching outside themselves to prove themselves consequential, usually in the mistaken belief that external achievement will establish their value. If not, why would they spend their lives seeking a place in the public's heart? Men like these are particularly broken, living as they do just one failure away from obscurity. They know that their value as human beings rests entirely in other people's hands. And they live in permanent and painful insecurity. They constantly question their self-worth and they turn to women both to feel desirable and sexy and to comfort them from their pain.

Yes, I know, men like Tiger Woods appear to the public as cool and collected. But beneath the calm veneer is a man who has been trained to believe that his value as a human being rests entirely on a never-ending game of human one-upmanship. Those who have made their names in the public sphere in realms like sports and politics live with unimaginable insecurity. And rather than deal with these insecurities in a healthy way by having deep emotional conversations with their wives about their fears, they find it easier to simply paper them over by turning to strangers who make them feel special. The attention of other women brings a momentary silencing of the inner demons that constantly taunt them with whispers of their own insignificance. And the more prized the woman is by other men, the greater the validation these men feel.

> In truth, men have affairs not for physical reasons but for emotional ones. They cheat not out of a sense of confidence but out of a state of brokenness. Not out of a sense of how desirable they are but out of a sense of what failures they are.

Coupled with this is the intuitive gravitation by men to the healing powers of the feminine. Men who are in pain use the caress and the care of a woman as a salve to soothe their broken egos. Having a woman care for you and make herself available to you – not to mention tell you how wonderful you are – becomes like a drug that makes you feel instantly better.

Of course, the healing is ephemeral and unfulfilling, based as it is on a highly artificial sense of intimacy.

The obvious question, now, is this: If a man who feels deeply insecure looks to a woman to make him feel special, then why doesn't he turn to his own wife? Why do husbands cheat on their wives and throw away their most important blessings? Why, when they have wives whom they cherish and who will do everything for them, is it still never enough?

The answer: Because any man who suspects deep down that he is a loser is going to look at the woman dumb enough to marry him as a loser squared. She has allied herself with failure and is part of the same loser package. By marrying someone with no value, however virtuous and accomplished she is in her own right, she has shown herself to be an even bigger loser than he is. Incredibly, the wife is unwittingly punished for her devotion. Men who feel like nothing see their families as impoverished extensions of their own nothingness. They require external validation to become a somebody. It takes the adoration of the crowds, the corner table in the restaurant, and the compliments of complete strangers to make a man like this feel unique.

And that's where you see great men becoming susceptible to affairs. It is specifically the woman to whom the powerful but insecure man is *not* married, the one who has not been devalued through a merger with failure, that can make him feel consequential.

Brian was a married man who made a good living as a lawyer. After being invited to speak at a conference for the first time, he fell in love with the feeling of adoration that came from the people who crowded around him after his speech. He became a sought-after speaker, but the conference organizers weren't the only ones seeking him. He started meeting women on his business trips. And he started sleeping with them. His marriage began to deteriorate. His wife did not know what he was up to, but she did know he accepted every invitation that came his way as if he never wished to be home.

They came to me for counseling and, with his wife out of the room, he confessed his numerous affairs. It took many sessions to explain to him that he was sleeping with women to gain a sense of personal validation, a diagnosis he resisted. "I am sleeping around because I am starved for sex," he insisted. "Then why aren't you have having sex with your wife?" I asked him. And while he gave some perfunctory reasons such as "she's not as attractive as she used to be," it was clear that he had no good answer other than this: the women he was not married to were the ones with the capacity to make him feel better about himself.

Egocentrism and narcissism are always the hallmark of the broken American male, who mistakenly believes that ephemeral attention is an adequate substitute for intimate love. This explains the steady stream of tragic stories that engulf so many powerful, accomplished, and popular men. Bill Clinton was the most powerful man in the world. But he still needed the ego boost of feeling desirable to a fawning, twenty-something intern. In truth, no amount of such validation would ever make these men feel like they matter because all the adulation is being pumped straight into a black hole. There is no bottom to these men's low self-esteem.

When money is made into a commodity for the purchase of self-worth, it requires an endless supply to make a dent.

And the same is true with power, fame, and women. Once you make a man's ego dependent not on the love he gets from his family but on the adoration he gets from crowds, he transfers the locus of his self-esteem away from his intimate circle and onto a fickle public. His need for public validation becomes an addiction. David Petraeus exhibited iron discipline in rising through the ranks of the toughest corporation of all, the US military. But that did not stop him from showing incurable weakness when a beautiful brunette made him feel like a hero. External accouterments, however grand, are always a poor substitute for authentic self-regard. Elliot Spitzer threw his career away with a high-class call girl. A woman who is so desirable that a night with her can set you back a thousand dollars can make a guy feel like a million bucks.

Former US Representative Anthony Weiner was back in the spotlight again with a mayoral run two years after having been forced to resign his seat in Congress in 2011 in the wake of a "sexting" scandal in which he sent lewd photos of himself to various women, even as his wife was expecting the couple's first child. "If you're looking for some kind of deep explanation, I simply don't have one," Weiner said to the press. "This was just me doing a dumb thing, doing it repeatedly and then lying about it."[60] But what would drive a man to seek emotional intimacy or erotic excitement with a woman other than his wife, over and over again? And why is it that we men don't seek deep answers within ourselves to this question, instead dismissing infidelity and dishonesty as "dumb" behavior? Remember that Weiner's indiscretions took place over the Internet and phone wires, not in person, so these weren't even physical relationships.

Many will argue with me: Adultery is about sex. It's about

powerful men behaving arrogantly. But then why is the most common refrain of the adulterous husband to his mistress the infamous "My wife doesn't understand me," meaning, *My wife can't take away my pain, but maybe you can. My wife can't make me feel good about myself. Even in my marriage I still feel so insignificant. But being with you makes me feel special.*

I was not at all surprised to hear Tiger Woods's alleged mistresses saying that he told them he loved them and was unhappy with his wife. Cheating husbands often say things like this. And at the time, they mean it. Monica Lewinsky said that Bill Clinton told her he would leave Hillary and marry her, which, whether accurate or not, is again common with the unfaithful spouse. They're expressing their inner misery and blaming their wives for their unhappiness when really they are solely responsible for their low self-esteem. Contrary to the cheating husband's fantasies of redemption in the arms of the other woman, the insecure overachieving man's brokenness will carry over into every relationship until he finally decides to fix himself.

Tuning In

Men think they want sex; they think they're programed by evolution to spread their genes, and that being a "sex addict" is a natural state of being for a red-blooded American male. Indeed, husbands often excuse their affairs by claiming to be sex addicts. I was once on a talk show where there was a man who professed to be a sex addict. So I went up to an attractive woman in the audience and I asked the sex addict, "Do you want to have sex with this woman?" He said, "Sure, of course!" I then turned to the woman's boyfriend, who was sitting with her. He was a big bodybuilder type. I said to him, "What would you do to this man if he laid a finger on your girlfriend?" He looked straight at the sex addict and said, "I would rip him limb from limb." I asked the sex addict, "Do you still want to have sex with her?" He shot back, "No, I think I'll pass!" I threw my hands up in the air and joyfully announced, "You're cured!" The addiction seemed to apply only when there was more pleasure than pain!

"Sex addiction" can often be used as a tawdry cover-up for a deeper problem. Current thinking is skeptical about this "disorder." A recent study headed by Nicole Prause, a researcher in the Department of Psychiatry at the Semel Institute for Neuroscience and Human Behavior at UCLA, dumps a bucket of cold water on the concept, finding no difference whatsoever in the brain responses of people who claim to be sex addicts versus those of non-"sufferers."[61] The condition is of such dubious status that the American Psychiatric Association did not include sex addiction in the updated DSM (Diagnostic and Statistical Manual of Mental Disorders), a catalog of all recognized psychological disorders. This is particularly revealing, since the DSM *is* willing to recognize disorders as trivial as "caffeine withdrawal."

The unacknowledged truth is that the male obsession with sex is in fact a deep-seated search for intimacy.

This is why we see philandering husbands so often having many mistresses, as opposed to just one. One study found that 46 percent of cheating men had multiple partners.[62] No woman can make a broken man feel good about himself. So he becomes a wanderer, obsessively traveling from woman to woman, hoping that at least one will provide the magical salve he seeks.

Many have said that husbands like Tiger Woods are sex

addicts. But if so, then why aren't they addicted to sex with their wives? Why does it have to come from another woman?

From understanding the cause we can cure the effect. Men who learn to talk to their wives about their deepest fears gain some measure of immunity against an affair. Infidelity, it turns out, often provides a starting point for couples to address the void in their relationship, which usually consists of the lack of truly intimate communication about life's anxieties and apprehensions. A man's deepest fear is of failure. And the person he most masks this from is his own wife, because she is the person whose opinion matters most. I know husbands who have been laid off from their jobs in this recession who still put on a suit every day and leave the house so that their wives won't find out. So-called "successful" men harbor the same fears. But rather than destructively address the fear by becoming a stud to other women, a man can purge from himself a dependency on strangers by learning to confide fully in his wife.

Men and women both live with tremendous pressures in our world. The difference is women talk about the pressures with each other. Guys rarely talk. Men may even see endless talking as juvenile and immature.

A friend of mine, married only two years, shared how his wife had an affair. This revelation was followed by a week of e-mails begging me not to tell any of his family members, who were wondering why he was despondent (it goes without saying, I would never have even thought of doing so). We men can't face that kind of humiliation. Sometimes I fear that for men, image is more important than heart.

You have to have an emotional outlet for pain. Married men should realize that they have in their wives everything they need, if only they would focus on bettering the relationship.

The number one complaint of wives in marriage is that their husbands don't talk to them about their feelings. When a philandering husband is trying to win his wife back after cheating on her, what better way than to finally open up to her about the reasons for his unfaithfulness? It was never a rejection of her. It did not happen because she did not give him enough sex, or because she didn't go to the gym, or wasn't emotionally available. Those are the excuses of a coward. A boy blames others for his failures. A man takes responsibility for his actions. Rather, it was because he falsely thought that someone other than his wife could make him feel good about himself. And now he has learned that those feelings of self-confidence are the preserve of only one woman.

> You have to have an emotional outlet for pain. Married men should realize that they have in their wives everything they need.

Through exploring the true intimate potential of the marital relationship, men can heal themselves and become true partners to their wives. But this kind of complete relationship can only happen when men stop turning their lustful attention outside the marriage. This means not only saying no to full-out infidelity but also not allowing sexual and emotional attention to be focused on other women in more "innocent" ways: no more Facebook affairs, no more pornography, no more flirting with women at work.

A man may excuse himself for being focused on other women with the common complaint that his wife has "lost interest in sex," almost a mantra in the American marriage.

Men need to think more deeply into *why* their wives seem to shut off intimacy.

> *Randy complained constantly that his wife was not interested in sex. Even when she was interested, to his mind it was very "vanilla": bland, no experimentation, missionary position only. "She won't let me tie her up," he told me. "She freaks out." I told Randy that in my experience as a counselor, without getting involved in his particular tastes, I had never met a woman who was not interested in sex. I had met many women whose husbands had never aroused them to the point where they would have any real interest.*
>
> *"If you don't take the time to heat up the oven," I told him, "don't complain when the dish is half baked."*
>
> *A woman's sexuality involves a process of arousal that Randy was not tapping into. Not only did he not compliment her, he in fact constantly made his wife feel bad; he would put her down, telling her he was much more sexual than she was. To deny someone's sexuality is to deny his or her essential humanity: what you're really saying is that this person is incapable of passion. I asked Randy to think about how he might have subconsciously contributed to this dynamic. "When was the last time you pursued your wife as you did before you were married?" I asked him. "You may feel that she no longer makes an effort to be attractive for you, but when was the last time you bought her jewelry or perfume or beautiful clothing? Have you made her feel that you notice her beauty? When she models new clothes for you or makes an effort to get dressed up to go out, do you compliment her? Do you make her feel desired?"*
>
> *I advised Randy to stop making his criticisms into a self-fulfilling prophecy. "Do the opposite," I suggested. "Compliment*

her, tell her she's beautiful, sultry, sexy. And you'll see her come alive." And that's what happened – their sex life went well beyond vanilla. But it did go into a lull at one point when he went into the same destructive patterns. Healthy eroticism isn't something where you can put in the effort a couple of times and expect to reap the benefits forever; it's an ongoing relationship that needs constant tending.

Sometimes it's the man himself who has no libido. Many people are depressed. Healthy sexuality is linked to self-confidence, and libido goes way down when people are not feeling good about themselves. (In addition, the very remedy for depression can also sometimes cause loss of sexual desire: many commonly used antidepressants have been linked to suppression of libido, and one in ten Americans over age 12 is on antidepressants.[63]) As we discussed above, a lot of men feel alone and isolated. Our society conditions men to feel bad about themselves. Everything is judged by material standards and one's position on the ladder of success. A lot of people reach a certain age and feel like their hopes and dreams have been crushed. They begin to lose faith in themselves. And men don't want to tell their wives how they're feeling, for a number of reasons: they don't want to appear weak; they don't want to appear unmasculine; they're not sure that their wives can offer any real comfort; they don't want to be pitied. Men want to pull themselves up by their own bootstraps. They also don't want to acknowledge their negative self-image.

> If you don't take the time to heat up the oven, don't complain when the dish is half baked.

This leads to a self-fulfilling, repeating cycle. The more

men shut their wives out, the more there's distance in the relationship, the more there's cause for depression, the more the libido sinks... It's a terrible negative feedback loop. A lot of these men turn to numbing agents – notably alcohol and television.

Kevin was recruited by his father, Raymond, to come into the family business. Raymond was looking to retire soon, and he wanted to leave his business in his son's hands. Raymond expected Kevin to grow the business and gradually take on more responsibility in preparation for Raymond's retirement. Kevin worked hard, but frankly he did not have much of a head for business and he never quite got the hang of it. He did a decent job, but not only did the business not grow, it kind of retracted under him. Raymond began to semi-retire, leaving Kevin with more and more responsibility for the day-to-day operations and long-term vision of the company. Raymond, who wanted to bow out, was too polite to take his son aside and tell him, "Listen, you're not the best at this... " It became the elephant in the room, the topic that neither could broach. Kevin felt like he was letting his father down, and even worse, he had no one to talk to about it. He sunk more and more into himself, feeling like he was a failure. He began to distance himself from his wife, Diane.

By the time Diane spoke to me about this, she and Kevin were having sex about once a month. Diane kept saying to Kevin, "Am I ugly? Did I become fat? Why won't you even touch me?" Kevin was in tremendous pain at his feelings of insignificance, worthlessness, and failure. But he couldn't tell her, because he couldn't acknowledge the dark space he had entered into, fearing that would make him feel even worse about himself. It was bad enough that he was doing poorly professionally; he didn't want to do poorly personally. So he just numbed himself with television. He would watch hours and hours of TV. Diane would go to sleep before him. And that's how their marriage proceeded, with emotional and sexual distance. She would ask him what was wrong and he would give the typical avoidant male response: "Nothing." I had to train Kevin to slowly begin to speak to his wife, with real baby steps.

What Kevin didn't realize was that by shutting Diane out, he was causing her tremendous pain. And even more than that, by refusing to share his feelings with his wife, he was depriving himself of emotional nourishment that could have held the key to surmounting his own pain.

Many men are suffering when they could be experiencing the balm and salve of their wives' loving attention. Sometimes, however, it must be said that wives can themselves contribute heavily to their husbands' distance. When a wife is not sympathetic, when she does not meet her husband's erotic pursuit with feminine nurturing, the balance of the relationship can become sadly disturbed.

Greg, an influential man with a lucrative job in banking, confided in me that his marriage was not doing well. He wanted me to speak to his wife separately and see if I could help resolve the gulf that had formed between them. Tracey minced no words when we met. "I really believe that Greg is gay. He doesn't touch me. We have almost no sex. I'm sure it's because he's gay." Tracey wanted children, making their disaffection even more painful. Tracey was so distraught over her husband's lack of interest in her – and so convinced of the cause – that she forced him to go to a psychiatrist to examine his latent homoerotic tendencies.

When I met later with Greg, he told a different story. He swore to me that he was straight. "Then why aren't you attracted to your wife?" I asked him. "Because she puts me down constantly," he said. "She's not nurturing at all. She's cold and punishing. She has a lot of anger issues she's never dealt with, and she really takes it all out on me."

I initially tended to side with Tracey. She was a very beautiful woman – always dressed beautifully, kept herself in shape. But the more I listened to her complain about him to me, the more I saw that there was a lot of truth to what he said. She was indeed a very angry woman, with a lot of unresolved anger from her childhood, and she had expected Greg to solve this for her. She was actually furious at him for not fixing all her issues. She felt that within her marriage she was supposed to finally be happy, yet she wasn't, so she blamed him.

Toxicity is a libido killer. Greg's lust for his wife had disappeared along with her femininity toward him. Sexual polarity had vanished and with it the feverish gravitation a husband should have toward his wife. In the end Greg and Tracey divorced. Greg married someone else and was very happy. But Tracey remained alone.

I have heard the same from many men, but I have heard it even more from wives. Countless married women have told me they are not attracted to their husbands because of how poorly they are treated. Sex is a chore rather than a pleasure. They have been turned off by their husbands.

Disconnectedness in a marriage is a painful state to be in. But so often it is of our own making; too many marriages wither for lack of even the most basic maintenance. Sometimes even the most hopeless-looking case can be turned around fairly simply, just by investing the necessary effort in the right direction.

There is an old story about a man who came to his rabbi with bitter complaints about his wife. "She's mean and harsh and demanding," he lamented. "She serves me terrible food when she cooks at all. She does nothing but yell at me with a tongue like a shrew's. My life with her is a misery," moaned the man, "but I can't stand the scandal of a divorce. I hate to admit it, but I have actually been praying that she should die and leave me in peace." The wise rabbi had a novel suggestion. "You know," he told his unhappy congregant, "when you make a pledge to charity and then do not fulfill the pledge before Rosh Hashanah, it's known that those close to you are liable to die in heavenly retribution. Why don't you make a large pledge to the community charity fund, and then not pay it?" The unhappy husband, a wealthy man not renowned for his generosity to communal causes, was delighted with the suggestion and implemented it immediately. He publicly pledged a large amount to the communal coffers, and then refused all attempts to collect the donation.

Months passed and the man eagerly awaited his wife's demise, but she appeared healthier than ever. The man became nervous and went to see the rabbi. "Nothing is happening," he reported. "She doesn't even have the sniffles!" The rabbi stroked his beard. "The death of a loved one is meant to be a punishment. Perhaps," he said, "you should make some efforts to appear to love her so that the divine decree will seem just. You have to create some evidence for the heavenly angels who will carry out the decree. Give her some gifts, compliment her, that sort of thing." The anxious husband was mollified. He set out for his home with renewed hope, ready to do his part. On the way, he passed the jeweler's shop and stopped in to buy his wife a lovely bracelet. She received the gift with astonishment, as he had not given her anything in many years. That night she served him his favorite supper.

Time went on and the man continued to invest himself in the project of appearing to love his wife so she would be punished by heaven with death. He complimented her, bought her gifts, and showered her with attention. In turn she stopped speaking to him harshly and began to treat him as king of his palace. The months flew by in an ever happier whirlwind. Before he knew it, the man looked at the calendar and realized that it was almost Rosh Hashanah! He ran to the rabbi in a panic and told him he was terrified that something would happen to his lovely wife! "You don't want her to die?" asked the rabbi. "God forbid!" said the man. "We've never been more in love! She brings me infinite happiness." "In that case," said the sage, "you have no choice but to make good on your pledge!" The man paid his generous pledge, and the couple lived the proverbial happily ever after.

What magic might happen in your own marriage if you work to create evidence of your love for and attraction to your spouse? When you tune in to what you have right in your own home, instead of seeking distractions outside the marriage, you may find that your marriage is not as moribund as you think. What can you do to make your spouse come alive? How can you reignite the passionate spark that once burned between you? Could it be that turning "Not tonight, honey, I've got a headache" into "Kiss me, you fool" is as simple as turning on, tuning in, and *not* dropping out?

PART 2

Mystery: What We Need to Know about Lust

Chapter 4

What Is This Thing Called Lust?

A Definition

Although in the popular mind, "lust" is something dirty, forbidden, sinful, selfish, and sleazy, Merriam-Webster's defines it like this:

1. (obsolete) a: pleasure, delight
   b: personal inclination: wish
2. intense or unbridled sexual desire: lasciviousness
3. a: an intense longing: craving <a *lust* to succeed>
   b: enthusiasm, eagerness <admired his *lust* for life>

The negative association we have with the word is legitimate; the Oxford English Dictionary says the chief current use of the word is associated with "intense moral reprobation" and describes "libidinous desire, degrading animal passion." Since the turn of the first millennium, Christian theology's censuring attitude has permeated the word. But notice that the original meaning of the word was simply pleasure or delight (the Oxford English Dictionary lists as additional obsolete meanings appetite, relish, inclination, and vigor). And even today the word carries the additional sense not only of intense longing (as for success) but also of enthusiasm and eagerness. Think of a "lust for life" and you'll see how positive it can be.

It's an undeniably zesty word. And it's that zest that I want to help you rediscover in your marriage and in your life. But please note: the choice for a zestful life is not a choice for quiet comfort. Lust by its very nature is unsettling. To lust is to feel torn in half. So you have to choose: do you want to be comfortable or do you want to be excited? A lustful marriage is the exact opposite of the "settling down" concept of marriage. This is not for the faint of heart. It's for those who want to live life at the mountaintop. It's for those who believe that healthy risk taking can lead to substantial rewards. But it is also fraught with potential peril. It can backfire, leading a couple to become more distant rather than closer.

> Lust is the constant, electrifying yearning to be one – to be made whole – by the object of your desire.

Let's start with a general definition of lust: lust can be described as the constant, electrifying yearning to be one – to be made whole – by the object of your desire.

Lust is a powerful pleasure cycle – much stronger than love. Love is so much more benign by comparison. It has nothing of lust's potency. Lust is exciting, all-consuming, and even overwhelming. It's a magnetic pull, but it goes much deeper than that, tapping into something so primal in our psyche that it cannot in any way be suppressed.

In fact, lust is a primal force not just within us but within the entire world. Attraction is built into the very structure of the universe. The Standard Model of particle physics explains the electromagnetism that causes molecules to form. Atoms are made up of an equal number of positively and negatively charged particles; this balance neutralizes the electrical charge of an atom. What makes these neutrally charged particles stick together to form molecules, then? The positively charged protons of one atom are electromagnetically attracted to the negatively charged electrons of another, and this attraction is the basis of the formation of the molecules that make up all matter. In the same way that men are drawn to women and women to men, the attraction of polar opposites is expressed at the molecular level, and the existence of the physical structure of our world is completely dependent on this force. Lust, it seems, makes the world go round – or more fundamentally, it just plain makes the world!

Even at the subatomic level we see the importance of attraction. Protons, the positively charged particles in the nucleus of an atom, should by all rights repel each other and atoms should just fly apart. But one of the four fundamental forces in the universe, an attractive force called the strong force, overrides the repellant effect by "gluing" protons to neutrons to keep the nuclei of atoms together. The counterbalance to the strong force is the weak force, which changes particles from one type to another as needed in a process called beta decay. The sun's nuclear fusion is powered by the strong force, but the weak force keeps the reaction happening at a steady rate that ensures the longevity of the sun. Likewise, lust is the strong force. It's what powers the fire. It's what keeps people from flying apart. Love – though I don't mean to sell something so special short – is the weak force. It's needed to keep the combustion stable and long-lasting, but it is ten million times weaker than the strong force, and it can't keep a nucleus – or a couple – together by itself.

Scientists have documented that the entire universe is filled with a constant hum of electromagnetic radiation, left over from the creation of the universe. This cosmic microwave background radiation might be likened to an undercurrent of deep desire in the universe – perhaps a remnant of God's deep desire to create the universe or to create man. Desire is an underlying force in the very essence of the universe that you can tap into.

Like a nuclear chain reaction, lust can be either productive or destructive, depending how it is used. A controlled nuclear chain reaction can fuel a power plant and provide energy to sustain life. Yet the same subatomic process when it is rapidly unleashed can fuel an atomic blast that destroys everything in its path. Likewise lust within a marriage can be a life-giving, sustaining source of energy, while lust detonated in the form of adultery or even lesser forms of infidelity is one of the most destructive forces that can hit a relationship. Adultery attaches the subatomic power of lust to the wrong target, with devastating results.

But while lust for a third party can be disastrous, one of the requirements for the sustaining of lust, interestingly, is community. They say it takes a village to raise a child. Well, believe it or not, it also takes a village to sustain erotic attraction! Think about it: you don't want something that no one else wants. For example, let's say a neighborhood suddenly gets hot and real estate skyrockets in the area. It's other people's desire that creates your desire. We're all dependent on that. Desire is almost like a universal energy. When one person allows it to flow, then other people are brought along with it. There's no such thing as eroticism that exists outside a community.

Robert and Nancy had been dating for several months and, although they shared interests, Robert was beginning to see some character traits in Nancy that disturbed him. He resolved to break it off, but that very day, his good friend Louis said to him offhandedly, "Nancy's a great girl. If you ever decide to break up with her, let me know because I would love to take her out!" It was an odd thing for a friend to say and it upset Robert. Yet, Louis's interest in Nancy rekindled Robert's desire as his competitive side took over. Robert did not break up with Nancy, but continued the relationship and eventually married her. Years later, after a bitter divorce, Robert realized that part of the reason he had married Nancy was because Louis had expressed his interest in her. Just as you don't want something that no one else wants, you definitely want something that other people want…

Lust, as the constant yet elusive striving and yearning to be one with the object of your desire, is ultimately a very frustrating state. Unlike love, which leaves you warm and cuddly, lust leaves you profoundly agitated and anxious. Ultimately it causes as much concern as it does comfort, as much pain as pleasure. This is why people often renounce lust: it's not a pleasant emotion. It's electrifying but not pleasant. It's not about comfort; it's about hunger. I wrote at length in my book *Ten Conversations You Need to Have with Yourself* about embracing hunger instead of rushing to immediately satisfy every urge and desire, so typical of life in the West. Embracing the insatiability of lust is a totally new mindset. We in America are all about scratching the itch. You fall in love and get married in order to "settle down," to purge yourself of anxiety.

The irony, however, is that purging yourself of anxiety

takes all the edge off of lust. If lust ultimately stems from a deep desire for a sense of completion or oneness, then achieving that completeness puts an end to lust. Lust is only kept alive by the *lack* of a sense of completion. This is why lust and loneliness always go together. Ultimately, lust – the desire to find completion – is a response to the inherent human desire to avoid loneliness. That's why there are three different levels of lust, corresponding to the three levels of loneliness we discussed earlier.

1. Material lust. This is the basest form of lust, corresponding to the human desire to avoid the first level of loneliness, aloneness, which is easily remedied by distraction. Material lust can take the form of objectified lust for a person, such as by looking at pornographic images. There is no actual relationship here, just an impersonal desire. Also in this category is the lust for an object. This kind of lust doesn't actually fire the erotic imagination. It triggers a deep yearning to have something and a feeling that you can't live without it, that you are incomplete without that object. People who lust after objects often try to incorporate these objects into their very being: look at the way people take care of an iPhone. They buy beautiful cases for them, nurture them like babies, make sure they never get scratched. I actually counseled a couple that had a huge fight because the wife dropped her husband's smart phone and cracked it; the husband went ballistic, as if the core of his being had been attacked. Lust for an object is ultimately a fraudulent form of connection.

Seeking completeness through an object (or a depersonalized, objectified connection such as looking at pornography) is of course an exercise doomed to failure. No object will ever complete you. This kind of lust will forever remain unsatisfied and unsatisfying. Sometimes we use material lust to compensate for emotional absence. Millicent Hearst, the wife of William Randolph Hearst, describes how, to placate her anger over her husband's affair with the actress Marion Davies, she went out and bought the most expensive pearl necklace in all of New York.[64] This is why people in the grips of material lust are forever lusting after a new object or a new partner: as soon as they have the object of their desire, they become disenchanted with it and look for the next one. Material lust is the type that gives lust a bad name. Ultimately it's a selfish indulgence.

2. *Emotional lust.* This level of lust corresponds to the human desire to avoid classical loneliness, the feeling of not being needed, which is remedied by being in an intimate relationship where someone else places you at the center of his or her existence. Emotional lust is a mental-psychological state of desire, characterized by the electrifying and intuitive gravitation of one energy to its polar opposite. True erotic desire falls into this category. The masculine and the feminine feverishly gravitate toward each other. This kind of lust can be tremendously rewarding and the source of a rich and profound connection, when it involves a loving relationship with your spouse. Emotional lust opens the door to the possibility of real intimacy in a relationship of mutual need: two people need each other, disclose the contents of their hearts to each other, and offer each other understanding and deep union.

3. *Spiritual lust.* Spiritual lust corresponds to the human desire to avoid the feeling that no one understands you, that you're alone in your pain and no one can reach you. Mystical-spiritual lust is the lust for God. A desire to become one with God is at the root of all deep spiritual experience. The

only being we can have total communion with is God. God is the One Being Who can truly understand your pain. That's why prayer is a psychological necessity: only deep communion with God addresses this need. Yet even the most spiritual person is left in a state of perpetual yearning, because we are prevented from complete union with God by our physical existence. So long as we have material existence in this world, our spirituality consists of the never completely fulfilled yearning to unite with God. Yet there is a physical outlet for this type of lust, as husbands and wives can have mystical-spiritual lust for each other, the two halves of one united soul seeking each other in a profound and deeply spiritual connection that is rooted in physicality and yet goes way beyond it.

All three of these types of lust have in common the desire to be completed, to find union – through an object (or objectified relationship), through an intimate relationship, or through the communion of souls. Lust is, inherently, a state of being unsatisfied, of *not having*. Once you have the object of your desire, lust has a tendency to evaporate. As overwhelming as lust is, it can also be ephemeral, raging one moment and spent the next. It's combustible. Lacking the proper fuel, it can sputter and die out. To keep lust alive, we have to understand it; we have to learn what those necessary conditions are.

We can learn a great deal by analyzing the conclusions of someone who was an accomplished student of lust. Steve Jobs was one of the greatest marketing experts in world history. What was his secret? It wasn't just Apple's technology, because there are other corporations with great technology. Steve Jobs understood that you can make people feel a hunger for and a yearning to be made whole by a product. He divined the secret of lust as an underlying force in the universe. He realized that if you correctly apply the principles of lust, you can superimpose it onto anything. This kind of material lust isn't a lust that fires the erotic imagination, but it creates within you a deep yearning to have something, a feeling that you cannot live without it.

Jobs, whose unwed birth parents gave him up for adoption on condition that the adoptive parents would send him to college, dropped out of Reed College in 1973 and traveled to India on a quest for spiritual enlightenment. His study of Eastern religions led to his understanding that sexual energy is the animating force of life. And Jobs set out to master lust.

Apple became the most valuable company in the history of the world because Steve Jobs saw that he could make people lust after his products. He could get them to wait in line for hours just to have them. He could have consumers hungering after a phone the way a man lusts after a woman and a woman after a man. He was the first marketer to really understand that his role was to make people not just want but actually *covet* his products.

Other companies may have good technology, and often at more competitive prices. But people don't wait ten hours on line to buy the other companies' phones. People camp overnight to buy an iPhone, because Jobs understood that lust is created through a specific set of principles that can be applied to nearly anything at any time. Jobs discerned the three principles of lust that we're going to explore in depth in this book.

The Three Principles of Lust

I. UNAVAILABILITY

Unavailability means frustrated desire, the inability to quench your longing. It's what relationships experts call "the erotic obstacle," meaning that something stands in between you and the object of your lust.

The first thing Jobs did with the iPhone and the iPad was to make them nearly impossible to buy. If you didn't get there by at least 6 a.m. to stand on line for a few hours when they were launched, forget it – you couldn't get one. They were gone in an hour, leading to lines stretching around the block in the sweltering summer heat. I personally witnessed hundreds of people baking in the New York sun in July 2008 when the iPhone 3G was introduced. Apple had to send out bottled water to prevent customers from fainting. People just had to have the phone. Tourists would give up whole days of their trips just to stand on line to get one. It was reminiscent of Cyrano de Bergerac waiting outside for Roxane, or Romeo hungering at the foot of the balcony of Juliet.

Now, who ever heard of a company that makes a product you can't buy? It goes against every principle of marketing. If you go into other electronics stores, there are mounds of product stocked up on shelves. And that's the whole point. They're stacked up because nobody wants them. Jobs did something counterintuitive. He made obstacles to purchasing his phone.

Love is always about constant availability; friendship is about familiarity, availability. Your wife or husband is your best friend, always there by your side: night after night, you've got sex on tap, whenever you want. (And somehow, more often than not, you don't want!)

Lust is about *unavailability*. After all, how can you lust after something that satiates your desire? If lust is the longing for something you can't have, then its consummation spells the immediate end of lust, no? Once you have the object of your desire, you no longer desire it. So should we take it to

> Lust is the longing for something you can't have. Once you have it, you no longer desire it.

an extreme and argue for *platonic* relationships where you're constantly in a state of desire? Let's not be ridiculous. No one wants to live in a relationship that is a perpetual tease without consummation. But the point is well taken: in order to keep on wanting something, there has to be some unavailability. That's the first principle of lust.

2. MYSTERY

The second ingredient of lust that Jobs discerned was likewise a strategy opposite that of nearly every other company: mystery and hiddenness. Jobs refused to release even an iota of information about the products he was developing before they actually dropped. He would not even acknowledge that certain products were in the pipeline, leading to constant speculation and a media frenzy to get any morsel about the product. Apple wouldn't even tell the press what product they were going to launch. They'd just say, "Come to an Apple event."

It's so counterintuitive. Don't you want to excite people about the product? Talk about it for months, even years, in advance, tell everyone how amazing it's going to be? Boeing announces the aircraft they're developing some half a decade before they roll out the actual product. They may have good reason to: they want to take advance orders. But even so, it impedes lust.

The reason why mystery is essential to lust is that curiosity is the soul of life. What does it mean to be alive? To be alive is to be a seeker, to be a knower: to want to know is the essence of sexuality and it's the essence of life itself. The only word the Bible uses to describe sex is *yediah*, knowledge.

> Lust thrives in mystery and disappears when there is too much light.

Western sexuality is today in a state of crisis. We see this in high divorce rates, in the degradation of sexuality through pornography and tasteless displays, in the dissatisfaction of married men and especially married women, and in the dearth of sex in marriage.

The sexual revolution was supposed to bring liberation, yet it has only brought dysfunction. Here's one of the principle reasons: Western sexuality is not based on knowledge. It's not based on seeking to know someone. We treat sex as a hormonal process – we're not looking to experience someone in the deepest possible way. We're rather looking to vent our hormonal buildup so that we can have peace.

Seeking knowledge is a profoundly unsettling journey. Why unsettling? Two reasons: First, when you seek to know something and have its mysteries revealed to you, the thing you seek has mastery over you. It causes you to have to acknowledge your own ignorance. The second reason it's unsettling is that you have no idea what you are going to discover. In that quest for adventure lies the soul of erotic longing: you are so mysteriously drawn to someone that you want to find out every last thing about him or her. And ultimately, carnal interaction goes beyond just speaking and knowing someone verbally and emotionally: it's to *experience* the person. That kind of intensity is unsettling and sometimes even frightening.

And therein lies the contemporary problem, because the essence of Western sexuality is to *never* be unsettled. The essence of Western sexuality is, on the contrary, the idea that hormonal buildup leaves you sexually frustrated, which is uncomfortable, so you either masturbate or you have sex. Western sexuality is about rejecting the discomfort of longing. You want to purge the urge, scratch the itch. And the idea is that you do it *in order to find contentment*. You feel discontented before sex. The purpose of the sexual encounter is to end the hunger. That's why orgasm is so central to Western sexuality. You engage in sex in order to achieve climax, which is radically different from Eastern practices of sexuality, like Tantra. What kind of mystery, what kind of quest for knowledge can exist in a relationship whose entire purpose is to *end* the quest for knowledge?

That's why sex dies off so quickly in a marriage. Think about it: it's simple, logical. If the point of sex is simply to satisfy a hunger, then after a year, two years, three years, how much hunger is left after eating the same dinner every night? Pretty soon you're going to want to start going to restaurants. It's a total bore.

But when sex is based on mystery, it's a completely different dynamic. You're not having sex because of a buildup of hormonal urges, not because you're trying to scratch an itch, but rather because you want to know this person deeply and intimately. You realize that your spouse has infinite layers that can be uncovered, one after the other, especially erotically. Sex is not a destination and you're not rushing to the finish line. It's rather an erotic journey of exploration. When you are means oriented instead of goal oriented, the possibilities are endless.

And here's why the erotic mind is so interesting: we've probably put more footsteps on the moon than we have on the erotic mind. It seems utterly mysterious to us. We don't even really understand eroticism, because the nature of the erotic mind is, to borrow a phrase from Freud, that it is "more powerful the less [it can] be expressed in words."[65]

Husbands and wives who really love each other are constantly probing and digging to find out secrets of their spouses' erotic minds, and these conversations can create lust. As we try to peel away some of the layers that conceal the mystery of our spouses' sexuality, we create great hunger and desire. Part of the purpose of this book – and of marriage itself – is to create opportunities that spark those conversations, some of them conventional and some of them highly unconventional.

The attraction of erotic mystery is universal. That's the reason why F. Scott Fitzgerald's 1925 novel *The Great Gatsby* is so successful and timeless: it taps into such eternal themes. Gatsby loses touch with his girlfriend Daisy and she marries someone else. That's one powerful erotic obstacle. When he learns that she lives across the bay and that the mysterious green light he can see from his home is actually emanating from hers, all of his longing for her is focused into that famous green light. It's so close yet also so distant, so pregnant with possibility, so utterly beyond his reach. There is also the sinful dimension: he wanted to marry her but she married someone else and now their relationship is completely forbidden.

The mystery that inspires lust is the possibility of exploration, of depths to plumb. This is part of the appeal of what

Steve Jobs offered: a communication tool that lets you delve into everything that's happening in the world, making you feel part of a larger community. With your smart phone you can text your friends and research anything you want and you have the illusion of completion. Of course, it's all virtual, and that's why he could introduce a new product every year and people would junk the old product upon which they had thought they were so dependent for the new one. As much as you try to fill a deep need with a piece of technology, ultimately it's so thoroughly unsatisfying that you feel the need to replace it, thinking, *oh, the next one is finally gonna do it for me!* That's horizontal renewal, a surface-deep exploration that feeds on an artificial sense of newness.

There's an alternative to this kind of superficial exploration. Instead of horizontal renewal, you can pursue vertical renewal. Instead of replacing your spouse, you can strive to go deeper and deeper in discovering his or her mysteries. That's how marriages stay passionate – when you believe there's still so much to discover and uncover about your spouse. And that's why keeping things a bit mysterious is one of the keys to keeping things alive and vital.

3. SINFULNESS

The third thing Steve Jobs discerned about the principles of lust is this: desire is magnified by sinfulness and forbidden-ness.

Jobs positioned Apple as the countercultural company that goes up against the dominant mainstream players like IBM. He gave Apple an air of rebelliousness. One of Apple's most successful slogans was "Think different." And they also produced what is regarded as the most influential TV advertisement of all time with their 1984 Big Brother ad, portraying IBM as a dominant, persecutory company that snuffs out individualism and color, leaving everything grey and monolithic. The ad, first aired during the Super Bowl the year George Orwell's anti-totalitarian novel *1984* caught up to its name, depicted rows upon rows of drably dressed people, their heads shaved, stripped of any individuality, listening to a "Big Brother" type on a giant screen declaiming about "the first glorious anniversary of the Information Purification Directives." A lone runner, brightly dressed in orange shorts and a white tank top featuring the Apple logo, carries a hammer which, despite being pursued by helmeted "thought police" types, she manages to hurl at the screen, destroying it in a dazzling explosion.

Apple portrayed itself as the subversive underground company that operates in the shadows to bust the monopoly. Apple was mysterious, rebellious, sinful, and did all the forbidden things. They shook up the industry and refused to play by the rules, thereby tapping into the third rule of lust, which is sinfulness. You want to see what you're not supposed to see, to have what you're not supposed to have. The very fact that something is off limits, that it goes against the rules, makes it enticing.

Imagine the following scenario. You go to a dance club, where you spend the entire evening engaged in a delicious flirtation with an attractive woman. You're speaking to each other, dancing together. She's indicating an interest in you. You're trying to win her over all throughout the evening: maybe you'll be able to conquer her and get her to come home with you. At a certain moment, when things are reaching a high pitch, she sidles up close to you and whispers in your ear, with her huskiest voice, "I can go home with you for a hundred bucks."

Bam, the eroticism is gone. The realization that she is only in it for the money instantly kills all erotic attraction. It turns out there was nothing forbidden about her – she was totally available from the very beginning. The moment you discover that, all attraction is lost. As they say, "Forget about her – she's a pro." As long as you thought you had to conquer her natural resistance, she looked like a prize to be won. The realization that she does not consider herself off-limits in any way but on the contrary is available to the highest bidder is deflating, to say the least.

Sinfulness is at the core of lust and eroticism because getting someone to sin for you is the ultimate form of validation. If you can get someone to do something sinful, that means that your attractiveness is so great that someone is prepared to overcome this highest of all obstacles – to do something that violates conscience, value systems, and even self-identity, *for you.* That's how desirable you are. That's how special you are.

That's why sin is so erotic. If you can get someone to contravene his or her own value system just to be with you – to sleep with you outside of marriage, or even to cheat on a spouse for you, that is the ultimate validation of your magnetism. If lust is a desire for a form of completion, then it has to be deeply complimentary in some way. For someone to be so out of control with desire for you that he or she is willing to abandon a value system, beliefs, and even bonds to other people, you have to be the most exciting, interesting person in the world.

To get what you're not supposed to have is the ultimate win: it raises you above the rules. It confers a special status on you. What's more erotic, a woman on the beach in a bikini, or a woman who has accidentally left the blinds in her bedroom open revealing her in skimpy underwear? They're both wearing the same amount of clothing, but the forbidden sight is so much more tantalizing. No matter how much flesh is exposed at the beach, you've been given license to see it and it's just not exciting. Sneaking a peak at what you are not supposed to see – getting a special privilege that comes with a thrill – that's erotic.

In the same way, it's the very legality of the marital relationship that robs it of lust. It's specifically the person who is forbidden to you that you lust after. And that's why Sir James Goldsmith famously said that when a man marries his mistress, he leaves a vacancy. Unfaithful husbands rarely marry the "other woman." There is no way to have exact statistics on this, but "it doesn't happen very often," according to Emily M. Brown, LCSW, director of Key Bridge Therapy and Mediation Center in Arlington, Virginia.[66] But even when men do marry their mistresses, such marriages are very unlikely to last. Australian golfer Greg Norman left his first wife for Wimbledon tennis champ Chris Evert, but divorced her fifteen months later to marry still another woman he'd previously had an affair with. I once counseled a man who married his mistress and then ended up leaving her within the first year of marriage.

When you think about the sacrifices a man would have to make to marry a mistress, it's astonishing that any man would ever be willing to give up a woman he fought so hard for. He has to get divorced, he alienates his wife and often the mother of his children, he may lose 50 percent of his assets, engage in ugly legal and custody battles, perhaps lose the affection of his children who now no longer respect him (no one likes to see their mother treated like a doormat)… all for this one woman, whom he often as not discards within a few years! Why does he no longer want her despite all he has gone through in order to have her? Simple: she's no longer forbidden to him! With the loss of all three rules of lust (she's no longer unavailable, she's no longer mysterious, and she's no longer sinful), lust is transformed to love and it's just not as strong.

Psychologist Jill Curtis, author of *How to Get Married… Again: A Guide to Second Weddings* (London: Hodder and Stoughton, 2003), says the same lack of luster is true for the mistress-turned-wife: "If the romance has been about a secret and a thrill, then the letdown after marriage may feel as if something has gone very wrong. After the passion of a secret affair, and then the wonder of whether he'll choose you, it can be hard to be with the man of your dreams all the time."[67]

> It's the person who is forbidden to you that you lust after, which is why even marriages need a sinful component.

As it says in Proverbs 9:17, "Stolen water is sweet." If you're not supposed to have it, boy, do you want it!

Is There Hope for Lust in Marriage?

As Steve Jobs so presciently understood, the three principles of lust – unavailability, mystery, and sinfulness – can be used to create lust for anything, and the presence of these three principles is vital to maintaining lust.

But wait: marriage seems to intrinsically involve availability, familiarity, and legality – the exact opposite of the qualities necessary to inspire lust! So how can lust survive marriage? Is there a way to maintain lust within the framework of a legally permitted relationship with someone who becomes more and more known to you over time and who seems to be constantly available? Is there any hope?

A married couple does have to share all the practical details of their lives, after all, so how do they carve out a space to know each other only in their essence? The cliché answer is to establish date nights, weekend getaways, "function-free zones" where after a certain hour of the evening you cease all talk of bills and so on. But the real answer is that you have to maintain your intimate relationship through the three principles of lust at all times, not just focus on it once every six months in a hotel. Love is the key to the stability of a marriage, but there has to be a constant undercurrent of lust.

When you call your wife in the middle of the day to say "I am calling you for no other reason than that I cannot get my mind off you," you are engendering lust. When you call and offer to take the kids to the dentist, you're engendering love. Love is practical; it's a partnership. Lust is a force that can't be denied or suppressed – I'm calling because I can't *not* call. When you take your wife shopping for beautiful clothing, that's lust. When you just give her the money to go shopping by herself, that's love. The lustful husband says "I want to *see* you in this."

And therein lies the key: your level of interest. Love is a calm partnership. Two people can sit cozily, each reading a different book, and the companionable feeling is sweet, but there's not much interest in it. Lust is a raging fire. People who lust for each other are entwined, engaged, and deeply drawn. When you are interested, you will want to fuel the fire. Exploring, building, and maintaining the three principles of lust is the key.

Chapter 5

The Unappreciated Treasure: Why We Shun Lust

We've looked at the reasons why marriage is faltering. We've looked at how our intimate disconnection affects women and men. And we've seen that American marriages are crying out for a good dose of passion. But why are we so resistant to this? If lust is so important, then why is it barely emphasized in marriage? On the contrary, the mere mention of it conjures up something sleazy in people's minds. Marriage should be noble, we think. We're above mere physicality. Get your mind out of the gutter. Right? We don't even recognize that something is missing! So the first step in revitalizing our moribund marriages is to understand why we not only don't prioritize lust but actually view it negatively.

In this chapter we're going to discuss the three reasons why we do not build marriage on lust today. Get ready for some myth-busting.

We Believe Lust Is Transient

Lust is seen as something unsustainable. It comes and it goes. It's flighty. We have been deeply socialized to believe that lust is a base chemical attraction that will inevitably fade with time. This is perfectly illustrated by a definition of lust found on the pop-culture website www.urbandictionary.com: "Often confused with love, [lust] is purely physical attraction and has no lasting effect." That's what we think of lust.

Hurricane Sandy hit the whole New York-New Jersey area and caused terrible devastation. Telephone wires and electrical cables were all blown away. A hurricane like that is more powerful than all the infrastructure; it's a force that cannot be resisted. But hurricanes don't come every day, and you rely on the infrastructure the rest of the time. So we rely on the infrastructure of love (the institution of marriage) and we try to ignore the hurricane of lust that will pass through from time to time.

People need Eros in their lives. Yet the best we seem to be able to do to sustain it is to regularly change partners, enjoying what we see as the initial chemical phase of each relationship, using it up and throwing it away to move on to the next conquest. This is a deeply counterfeit and lazy version of lust.

Kimberly is a vivacious, attractive, bubbly, highly intelligent woman who wants to get married. At least, she says she wants to get married, but her criteria are pretty stiff. As Zsa Zsa Gabor apparently once said, "I want a man who's kind and understanding. Is that too much to ask of a millionaire?" Kimberly has her sights set on marrying a man of means, and she doesn't date guys who aren't highly successful. But somehow, even among the pool of super-rich guys she's dating, she'll be in a relationship for six weeks, maybe eight weeks, and it's over. Kimberly cannot allow herself to get past the initial excitement and drama of a new relationship. The minute she starts to get comfortable with someone and the natural drama of a new fling begins to calm down, she creates drama. She finds something to fight about, something to make a scene out of.

Basically, Kimberly is an adrenaline junkie. She fears boredom. But there's a deeper reason for what's happening to her. There are four stages in a romantic relationship: attraction (the mysterious and inexplicable "chemistry" between people), verbal exploration (basic communication), emotional intimacy (sharing secrets), physical intimacy (carnal desire). In a healthy relationship, these four stages are cumulative: each one is internalized before going on to the next, so that by the time physical intimacy occurs, it's a culmination of the previous three stages, all of which remain active. Internalizing and incorporating each of these stages in turn makes for a wholesome relationship that includes communication, emotional intimacy, and passion. What Kimberly is doing, however, is passing through these stages without incorporating them, so that each one begins, quickly runs its course, and ends, instead of becoming a permanent feature of the relationship. So by the time Kimberly gets physical with someone, the stages of the relationship are already over. There is no adventure left. There is nothing to look forward to and nothing to explore – her relationships become boring to her before she can ever progress to true intimacy.

Hollywood is full of examples of the "conquer and move on" phenomenon. Elizabeth Taylor married eight times, and so did Larry King. Billy Bob Thornton has married five times, and his ex Angelina Jolie has moved on to third husband Brad Pitt, himself divorced from Jennifer Aniston. Geena Davis and Liza Minelli each tied the knot four times, as did Frank

Sinatra and William Shatner. Hollywood pairings often call to mind that old maxim about the weather: "If you don't like it, just wait fifteen minutes and it'll change." This is not to pass judgment on the individuals involved but rather on a celebrity culture that seems to mark marriage as disposable.

Out in the "real world," musical chairs is a little less common, at least after tying the knot: as of 2009, 15 percent of all Americans over age 15 had married more than once.[68] But everyone has met people who skip out on romantic relationships as soon as the chemistry fades. An even more common scenario, however, is that people fall in love, enjoy the lusty early phase of their relationships, and then quietly accept what they consider the inevitable decline of the quality of their intimate relationship. Once the chemistry is gone, it's gone, according to this view: physical attraction is a tool to get relationships started, but it can't possibly be expected to last. Kids come along, the relationship shifts, people mature, they are busy and distracted, they get old. As the joke goes, the three stages of sex in marriage are triweekly, try weekly, and try weakly. That's just the way it is, according to the common wisdom: lust is destined to fade and die.

> As the joke goes, the three stages of sex in marriage are triweekly, try weekly, and try weakly. That's just the way it is, according to the common wisdom: lust is destined to fade and die.

We don't expect lust to be present after the initial phase of a relationship because we don't even think it's possible. We think lust inevitably dies out over time.

Brandon and Heather, a couple in their mid-thirties, had

been married thirteen years when I met them through mutual friends. After they heard that I wrote books, they read some of them. One day Heather called me up and said, "My husband and I are very happy – we have a great marriage. But I have to take issue with what you said in your book *Kosher Sex* about how sex is the lifeblood and the soul of marriage. We have sex about once a month, and it's just fine with us. We're very happy and we love each other very much." "You're not serious!" I said. Heather assured me that she was very serious. "Is that sufficient intimacy?" I asked. "Sex no more than twelve times a year?"

Heather told me that at the beginning of their relationship they had been tremendously drawn to each other. In the first year of their marriage, they couldn't keep their hands off each other – she claimed they had sex four or five times per day. Brandon had been a very lusty person and Heather, who had less sexual experience before marriage than Brandon did, found everything new and exciting. They were mutually enraptured and explored each other hungrily. After a while their first child was born and things died down a little bit, as they are wont to do. When their second child came along, Brandon and Heather's love life died down even more. They went from having sex four or five times a day to three times a week to once a week, and eventually, by the time I met them, to no more than once a month.

"We don't miss it," Heather said. We love our kids, we get along great, and we're very happy with things just the way they are. After all, we've been married thirteen years. That's just the way it goes after you're together for a while – passion wears off and you become good friends; you share this kind of comfortable closeness. It's only normal."

"This is abnormal," I protested. "Your sex life isn't a priority in your marriage at all?"

"Sure it is. I mean, we're very attracted to each other. It's just that we're very busy people," Heather said. "Between work and the kids and the house and our community obligations… we're just very tired. Who has energy for sex?"

"The whole reason you're tired is that you have no libido," I said. "You think that you have a libido but you're tired. No: you're tired because you have no libido. Your life force is drained."

Heather politely agreed to disagree, insisting that she and Brandon were very satisfied with their marriage and everything was just fine between them. I later heard that Heather and Brandon regretted meeting me, because before she had spoken with me they were blissfully happy. Now I had introduced doubt.

Some months later Heather called me again and asked to make an appointment for marriage counseling. I apologized for having upset her and said, "Maybe it's best that you not come to counseling. If your marriage is working for you as it is, then maybe it's better not to tamper with things. If a more active sex life isn't important to you, then it isn't important to you." Heather broke into tears.

She had been living fraudulently, she told me. She wasn't even a woman to her husband. There was no deep attraction, no deep connection. She was no longer sorry she had spoken with me, because rather than feeling I had betrayed her, she had come to feel that I had opened her eyes.

Opening your eyes can be very painful, and so it was in this case. During our sessions Brandon eventually confessed that he had for a long time been engaging in excessive *masturbation. But he had never admitted that to his wife: there were many secrets that were not being shared. When the veneer came down, it turned out that this "happy" sexless marriage was not so happy after all. Heather and Brandon had allowed their marriage to wither.*

Fortunately, Brandon and Heather were able to rebuild their relationship. But I wonder sometimes what would have happened if they had continued as they were: Would they have woken up one day after the kids had grown up and moved on, and realized that they were complete strangers to each other? How many more couples are living like roommates, never thinking that there is anything to be done about it, because they assume that the death of passion is the inevitable end of all long-term relationships?

One reason for this assumption is that we make the mistake of associating lust purely with the physical. We think it's centered in the body, and that as bodies get older and more tired, lust has to also fade. But this is a fundamental misconception. Lust, as we saw in Apple's marketing strategy, is not centered in the body: it's the gravitation of two energies – masculine and feminine – toward each other. It's a cosmic coming together of complementary forces, recognized by the Chinese as *yin* and *yang*, by the Hindus as *jivanmukta* (a person who has synthesized masculine and feminine), and by Kabbalah as *zeir anpin* and *nukvah* (masculine and feminine). Lust is much more in the mind and soul than in the body.

We Believe God Is Love and Lust Is Wrong

"Love is a many-splendored thing," crooned Frank Sinatra, and that's certainly how Western society sees it.

It is love that asks, that seeks, that knocks, that finds, and that is faithful to what it finds. (Augustine of Hippo)[69]

One word frees us of all the weight and pain of life: that word is love. (Sophocles)[70]

When love speaks, the voice of all the gods
Makes heaven drowsy with the harmony.
(William Shakespeare, *Love's Labour's Lost*)

Love is touted as the grandest, largest force in the universe. How could lust be more important than the romanticization of love? Love has dominated Western culture for two millennia, ever since John put quill to parchment and wrote, "Whoever does not love does not know God, because God is love" (1 John 4:8). Over and over again in the Christian Bible, the concept is repeated: "God is love. Whoever lives in love lives in God, and God in them" (1 John 4:16).

God is love, love is exalted holiness, and therefore, we believe, marriages should be based on love and certainly not on lust. The source of this view, however, is not the Hebrew Bible but the New Testament. You'll notice that in the Five Books of Moses (the Hebrew Bible), it doesn't say anywhere that God is love. That *God is the source of love*, and that *God loves*, certainly, but Judaism never says that God is so monolithic as to be described merely as love. God is not love. God is many things. The Jewish tradition would say that God is utterly beyond description. We can understand Him only indirectly, as for example through the ten kabbalistic *sefirot* (emanations) through which God interacts with the world. And likewise love is just one of the tools God uses to run the world.

The Kabbalah gives the following metaphorical

explanation of the nature of the God. Take water. It is colorless. But you can put it into any colored glass and it will look from the outside as if the color has changed. Thus, water in a red glass will look like it is red. But all the while, the water inside remains colorless. So too with God. He is utterly beyond description, infinite, colorless. And God uses ten channels, ten colors, if you will, called the *sefirot*, with which to interact with us. One of them is *chesed*, or love, compassion, benevolence. Another is *gevurah*: severity, stringency, judgment (think about God smiting the Egyptian firstborn or sending the waters of the split sea crashing down on Pharaoh and his soldiers). But God is neither love nor judgment. He is utterly beyond all description. Saying that God is love is limiting, and God is always infinite and unlimited.

In the Christian view, since God is love, love is the ultimate good: "Love is patient, love is kind. It does not envy, it does not boast, it is not proud. It is not rude, it is not self-seeking, it is not easily angered, it keeps no record of wrongs. Love does not delight in evil but rejoices with the truth. It always protects, always trusts, always hopes, always perseveres. Love never fails" (1 Corinthians 13:4–8). What a beautiful summary of the virtue of love – and its limitations! This is the perfect description of a model of love as companionship and friendship. And if anyone wants to have a romantic relationship based on these warm and cuddly attributes, that's admirable. Every marriage should be so lucky. But left to its own devices it's also a recipe for boredom and monotony.

Lust, by contrast, as one of the seven deadly sins, is disparaged in Christian tradition as something pornographic: "For everything in the world – the lust of the flesh, the lust of the eyes, and the pride of life – comes not from the Father but from the world" (1 John 2:16). Lust is ungodly; it does not come from God and apparently it even contradicts His will.

Indeed, the ultimate model held up for virtuous Christians is abstinence, with marital relations being merely a concession to human weakness. Paul explains in Corinthians:

> Now for the matters you wrote about: "It is good for a man not to have sexual relations with a woman." But since sexual immorality is occurring, each man should have sexual relations with his own wife, and each woman with her own husband. The husband should fulfill his marital duty to his wife, and likewise the wife to her husband. The wife does not have authority over her own body but yields it to her husband. In the same way, the husband does not have authority over his own body but yields it to his wife. Do not deprive each other except perhaps by mutual consent and for a time, so that you may devote yourselves to prayer. Then come together again so that Satan will not tempt you because of your lack of self-control. I say this as a concession, not as a command. I wish that all of you were as I am. But each of you has your own gift from God; one has this gift, another has that.
>
> Now to the unmarried and the widows I say: It is good for them to stay unmarried, as I do. But if they cannot control themselves, they should marry, for it is better to marry than to burn with passion. (1 Corinthians 7:1–9)

Sexuality, then, is to be managed, if absolutely necessary, through the marital relationship. But it would be better and more virtuous, in the Christian view, for people to live without sexuality if they are able to do so.

About ten years ago there was a case in Texas where a

woman named Joanne Webb was bringing in some extra money for her household by hosting Tupperware-style home "Passion Parties," selling "marital aids" – lingerie, sex toys, and the like – for married women. She was arrested under Texas indecency laws and her evangelical mega-church revoked her membership. So I invited her on my radio show. And I invited my friend Reverend Flip Benham from the pro-life Operation Rescue in North Carolina to be my foil and debate me.

During the show, I told Joanne that if she had been a member of a synagogue, she would probably have been given a medal! The rabbi would have said, "You're making women more attractive to their husbands? Mazel tov!"

Well, Reverend Benham was appalled. He wanted to know how I could applaud what this woman was doing. When I asked him what exactly was wrong with selling marital aids to married women, he said something along of the lines of, "Shmuley, she was trying to make men objectify and lust after their wives." So that was her crime: she was trying to increase lust in marriage! A man has to learn to respect, love, honor, and cherish his wife, said Reverend Benham, not degrade her with lust.

This is a deeply ingrained idea in Christian culture: lust is what a man feels when he looks at porn, what a woman feels when she is working out with her trainer while her husband is paying the bills. Lust is something we automatically assume is illicit, forbidden, selfish, denigrates the human condition, speaks to our basest human impulses.

Fortunately, the charges against Joanne Webb were eventually dropped, but the sentiments that caused the trouble for her in the first place are still very much alive. So many people in America, whether Christian or not, have absorbed this idea at a fundamental level: we don't bring lust into our marriages because we believe in the fiber of our beings that lust is simply *wrong*.

Just as Reverend Benham articulated, we believe that our marriages should be ennobled by love rather than degraded by lust. American drama critic and editor George Jean Nathan (1882–1958) captured this sentiment perfectly when he said, "A man reserves his true and deepest love not for the species of woman in whose company he finds himself electrified and enkindled, but for that one in whose company he may feel tenderly drowsy."[71]

> We don't bring lust into our marriages because we believe in the fiber of our beings that lust is simply *wrong*.

Being electrified and enkindled, apparently, is for the single man, and he doesn't love the women who inspire these feelings in him. A marriageable woman, on the other hand, is one who evokes feelings of virtuous tender drowsiness. Is this a recipe for satisfaction in the marital bedroom?

We Believe Lust Is Politically Incorrect

The modern couple has a relatively new piece of baggage to haul into that bedroom. Those raised in the 1960s or later have internalized a lot of messages that came out of the feminist movement. Today's culture of gender equality erases differences between the sexes, promotes sameness, and posits that it is wrong to "objectify" a woman as a sexual being.

President Obama himself found this out in a big way when in a Silicon Valley fundraising appearance he praised California Attorney General Kamal Harris's looks: "She is brilliant and she is dedicated and she is tough, and she is exactly what you'd want in anybody who is administering the law, and making sure that everybody is getting a fair shake," he said, and then followed up his remarks with the controversial bombshell: "She also happens to be, by far, the best-looking attorney general in the country."[72]

CNN ran an opinion piece that slammed the president, saying, "This is how you talk about a colleague, a fellow elected official, a fellow lawyer with the goods to compete head to head with any man in the country?"[73]

Note that Obama *first* praised Harris's intelligence, work ethic, character, and competence, and only then added a compliment about her physical appearance. Nevertheless Obama was forced to "eat crow" and issue an apology.[74]

There are still plenty of examples of women being treated as "window dressing" and being evaluated based on their looks rather than their accomplishments – often with a presumed inverse relationship between beauty and brains. Think Sarah Palin, who was frequently described as good-looking and simultaneously accused of intellectual inferiority.[75] One story on the topic of Palin's looks began, "Did Sarah Palin seduce influential Republicans with her looks?"[76]

Nevertheless, the "enlightened" segment of American society considers a woman's attractiveness to be an untouchable subject, and mandates identical treatment for men and women. "California's tough AG has fought stereotypes about her looks since the start of her career," scolded one article on the Obama-Harris kerfuffle. "Obama knows better."[77]

Noticing a woman's looks is sexist, as any good college-educated man knows. Furthermore, chivalry went out with the 78 rpm record. Post Gloria Steinem and Betty Friedan, opening a door for a woman became a crime of repression. In fact, the idea that men and women might be different in any way at all became anathema.

There has been some backlash against the idea that men and women are identical in every way except their biology. Beginning in the 1990s, social scientists began to publish books and studies suggesting that in fact some aspects of differing male and female behavior may be influenced by genetic factors.[78] It may be that the pendulum is swinging back in the direction of acknowledging that men and women are not identical. Nevertheless, many men and women today grew up internalizing a very strong taboo against the idea of gender differences, and above all against looking on a woman as a sexual being in any way. A man who lusts after a woman is viewed as a boor and an unevolved, low-class Neanderthal, the archetypal construction worker whistling at ladies walking past and being slapped with a sexual harassment suit.

Does a woman's sexuality in fact have any place in the board room? Should a man see his female coworker as a sexual object? Obviously, no one wants a situation where a man is seeing women only as sex objects and can never take a woman seriously as someone who has a mind. But ironically, taking it to the opposite extreme can get coworkers into some very compromising situations. Let's say a man and a woman work together in a company and they both have to travel on company business. If they do not acknowledge the possibility that they could be attracted to each other, and the woman is treated exactly the same way as her a male coworker, then they could save the company money by sharing a hotel room!

Not only is that inappropriate, but it's actually profoundly unflattering to a woman because it implies that she could never exert an attractive force on a man. Yet this is exactly what we do in society when we bend over too far backwards trying to avoid the sexist situation where a woman is devalued and seen only as a sex object. And this attitude is not limited to the public arena. Many people, especially highly educated people, are so convinced that seeing a woman as a sexual being devalues her that they end up in the mindset that it's simply not politically correct to have desire at all, even if the woman in question is your wife! As rabbi at Oxford University, I certainly saw this dynamic often enough.

> *Anthony and Carolyn were members of the L'Chaim Society I founded at Oxford University. They were the typical left-wing university types, very much into the Green Party and liberal causes. When they married, they both took each other's last names, combining them with a hyphen, as was the vogue then in their crowd. Anthony felt that the two of them were perfect soul mates. "We have the same politics," he said. "We like the same films. We have the same values." But I detected an unhappiness in Carolyn, and when I spoke with the two of them, Carolyn confessed that in fact something was missing for her in their marriage. She said it was true that they loved each other deeply, but then she said to her husband, "You're afraid to long for me as a woman. You feel it would be wrong of you to desire me." Although Carolyn appreciated their deep compatibility and companionship, in the deepest part of her she really wanted to be desired.*
>
> *Anthony was taken aback by Carolyn's politically incorrect admission. His response was, "I'm not an animal. I have worked to transcend that. Would you want me to be some guy that just beds you and doesn't respect you?" Anthony felt he was more enlightened and evolved than that: he would never*

debase his wife by lusting after her. When he and Carolyn made love, he wanted to have very slow, tender lovemaking that included a lot of talking. It was all very cerebral and gentle and civilized. But it turned out that what Carolyn was really craving was for him to sometimes just take her – passionately and with utter abandon – because he couldn't help himself.

Both the Christian idea and the academic idea that lust is degrading come from the same root: that it is love that is noble, while lust is lowly, carnal, and demeaning. Aristotle wrote, "The mass of mankind are evidently quite slavish in their tastes, preferring a life suitable to beasts.... [P]eople of superior refinement and of active disposition identify happiness with honour."[79] In short, the mind is good and the body is bad; the intellect is lofty and the primal drives are lowly. Lust is nothing but a bestial impulse that the noble person will surmount. This Aristotelian idea is firmly implanted in Christianity as well, and this hierarchical mind/body compartmentalization is the normative view in Western society.

In this context where natural desires are considered a lowly impulse that must be transcended, the very idea of sexual attraction is somewhat disparaged. It's almost as if the idea of people being physically attracted to each other were passé. So the third reason we shun lust in marriage is that we consider it unenlightened and politically incorrect.

It's almost as if the idea of people being physically attracted to each other were passé. We consider lust unenlightened and politically incorrect.

For all the reasons enumerated in this chapter, we've

internalized the idea that lust is a flash in the pan, a temporary moment of chemistry, and furthermore that it is immoral, animalistic, and essentially somewhat distasteful. Love, on the other hand, we see as worthy, solid, dependable, elevated. We think love is the only reasonable basis for a marriage.

But I have a surprise for you: the Hebrew Bible actually recommends the opposite.

Chapter 6

Cleaving: Love and Lust in the Hebrew Bible

The Holy of Holies

In contrast to the New Testament's emphasis on love in marriage, the Hebrew Bible recommends building marriage on a foundation of lust. Not only does it recommend this, in fact, it actually *commands* it. Don't believe me? Let's take a look. Twice in the Bible (Exodus 20:14 and Deuteronomy 5:18[80]), we are commanded in the last of the Ten Commandments: "You shall not covet your neighbor's wife." Now, think about this a minute. The direct implication is that you *should* be coveting your *own* wife. Because if lust and covetousness were wrong, the commandment would say you should not covet *any* woman. But it doesn't say that.

> The Tenth Commandment says, "You shall not covet your neighbor's wife." The direct implication is that you *should* be coveting your own wife. Because if lust and covetousness were wrong, the commandment would say you should not covet *any* woman.

You shouldn't have illicit lust but you should have holy lust. The Bible itself proclaims lust as holy. Exodus 38:8 relates that when the nascent Jewish nation constructed the Tabernacle and its implements in the wilderness, they "made the bronze basin and its bronze stand from the mirrors of the women who served at the entrance to the tent of meeting." The eleventh-century Jewish sage Rashi comments on this verse that Moses objected to melting down the women's copper mirrors to make implements for the holy Tabernacle. After all, these mirrors had been used for base purposes, to beautify the women and arouse their husbands' desire. This prompted a correction from God Himself, Who instructed Moses: *Kibel*, "Take them," *ki eilu chavivin alai min hakol*, "for these are dear to Me above all."[81]

During the time when Pharaoh had decreed a death sentence on any baby boy who would be born to the Hebrews, the husbands had separated from their wives, not wanting to produce children who would be born in such circumstances. The wives used their copper mirrors to arouse their husbands and conceive children in defiance of the decree. These mirrors were precious to God because the lust the women aroused in their husbands represented the ultimate embrace of life.

Although the copper basin was lost to us upon the destruction of the Holy Temple, the women's copper mirrors still receive a prominent place in the Jewish home, in the *charoset* (an apple mixture) that is placed on the Seder table, recalling the verse "Under the apple tree I roused you; there your mother conceived you" (Song of Songs 8:5).

The lust of a husband for his wife is beloved by God, enshrined in our holiest Scripture.

Perhaps the most vivid biblical proof of the exalted place of sexuality is the Bible's beautiful erotic love poem, Song of Solomon (also called Song of Songs). There are twenty-four books of the Hebrew Bible, and the Talmud says the holiest of them all is Song of Songs. The Talmud calls it *kodesh ha-kodashim*, "holy of holies."

Now, if you read it, you may be confused, because the entirety of the book is an erotic love poem about a man and a woman who lust after each other.

Jews primarily read the Song on the holiday of Passover, which celebrates the emancipation of the Jewish slaves from Egypt. Being freed of Egyptian slavery made our bodies free, but it did not necessarily make our spirits come alive. You can be freed from the slavery of Egypt but still be enslaved to the drudgery of everyday life; just because your body is free doesn't mean your heart is. The monotony of everyday existence is its own form of slavery. God wanted us not merely to exist, but to *live*; not just to get by with necessities, but with magic. And the Song of Songs is a guide to lifting your life out of the doldrums and into the heights of erotic yearning.

At first glance, the Song seems downright unbiblical. In fact, you might even wonder what this book is doing in the biblical canon. Just read some of the verses. You'll be scandalized. Here is but a sampling:

Let him kiss me with the kisses of his mouth – for your love is more delightful than wine. (1:2)

Your breasts are like two fawns, like twin fawns of a gazelle that browse among the lilies. (4:5)

Your stature is like that of the palm, and your breasts like clusters of fruit. I said, "I will climb the palm tree; I will take hold of its fruit." May your breasts be like clusters of grapes on the vine, the fragrance of your breath like apples, and your mouth like the best wine. (7:7–9)

Imagine a rabbi or priest reading these verses from the pulpit. That would raise some eyebrows, huh? Would kids even be allowed to listen?

And yet, not only is this very erotic poem in the Bible, but the ancient rabbis declared it to be the Bible's most sacred book. Rabbi Akiva, one of the greatest rabbis ever to live, declares: "The entire universe is unworthy of the day on which the Song of Songs was given to Israel. For all the books of the Bible are holy, but the Song of Songs is the holy of holies" (Mishnah *Yadayim* 3:5). Other sages quoted in Midrash Rabbah proclaim that Song of Songs means "the best of songs, the most of songs, the finest of songs."

The book's erotic nature has led many scholars to interpret it in allegorical terms. Some ancient scholars maintain that the Song describes the relationship not between two mortal beings, but between God and His people. Maimonides, the twelfth-century Jewish sage whom many consider the greatest rabbi of all time, understands the Song as an extended metaphor for the love of the individual pious soul for God.

The allegorical interpretations are valid, and no doubt the Song is pregnant with deep spiritual and mystical meaning. But it is still undeniable that, at its core, the Song is a highly erotic story captured in verse, and the Bible uses these deeply sensual descriptions to convey mystical insights. The Song celebrates a highly erotically charged relationship between a man and a woman. To dismiss this completely is to miss the central message of the Song. A rabbinic tradition teaches that no biblical verse ever loses its literal meaning.[82] The Song of

Solomon is an erotic poem; we need to know why the Bible would find it so holy.

Here's the secret of the Song and much else in life: God is a burning conflagration, a raging inferno, vibrancy itself. Moses encounters God in a burning bush. The Israelites are lead through the wilderness of Sinai by God represented as a pillar of fire. And in our relationship with God, indeed in our relationship with all things outside us, we need to find passion.

And herein lies the hidden secret of the Song, the foundation of Eros: never once in the poem are the lovers described as finally indulging their lust for each other. They live in a perpetual state of hunger. They never meet. Their desire is never consummated. They are always seeking and just missing each other. The lovers in Song of Songs perfectly encapsulate the principles of lust, beginning with rule 1, unavailability. They live in a state of frustrated desire:

> Here's the secret of the Song of Solomon and much else in life: God is a burning conflagration, a raging inferno, vibrancy itself. The human personality, created in the same image, yearns to burn with the same vitality: hence, our lifelong search for erotic passion.

> All night long on my bed I looked for the one my heart loves; I looked for him but did not find him. I will get up now and go about the city, through its streets and squares; I will search for the one my heart loves. So I looked for him but did not find him. The watchmen found me as they made their rounds in the city. "Have you seen the one my heart loves?" (Song of Songs 3: 1–3)

Lust is awakened through obstacles and absence. It is quieted through satiation and fulfillment. Lust is fundamentally about unfulfilled longing: it is a lonely emotion of night and shadow. It thrives in an atmosphere of separation and distance rather than comfortable familiarity.

The Song continues:

> I slept but my heart was awake. Listen! My beloved is knocking: "Open to me, my sister, my darling, my dove, my flawless one. My head is drenched with dew, my hair with the dampness of the night." I have taken off my robe – must I put it on again? I have washed my feet – must I soil them again? My beloved thrust his hand through the latch-opening; my heart began to pound for him. I arose to open for my beloved, and my hands dripped with myrrh, my fingers with flowing myrrh, on the handles of the bolt. I opened for my beloved, but my beloved had left; he was gone. My heart sank at his departure. I looked for him but did not find him. I called him but he did not answer. The watchmen found me as they made their rounds in the city. They beat me, they bruised me; they took away my cloak, those watchmen of the walls! Daughters of Jerusalem, I charge you – if you find my beloved, what will you tell him? Tell him I am faint with love.

Lust is lovesickness. It leaves us pining and empty rather than accomplished and fulfilled. It heightens our insecurities and magnifies our vulnerability. Lust creates an anxiety that rocks the foundation of our existence. To lust is to have no peace. It is to wander without finding, to seek without discovering, to thirst without drinking. Yet for all of that, nothing quite addresses our needs more profoundly or strikes deeper into the very core of the human personality.

In its most famous verse the Song says, "Many waters cannot quench love; rivers cannot sweep it away. If one were to give all the wealth of one's house for love, it would be utterly scorned" (8:7).

All the water in the world cannot put out the fires of lust. To lust after someone is to be invaded in mind, body, and spirit. It is to mentally anguish over having or seeing the object of one's lust. Married women who have affairs report being unable to focus on their children or even simply to do the dishes. They are permanently distracted. One woman told me, "Since starting this relationship my whole body tingles and I cannot sleep. I go through the night in a twilight zone between consciousness and sleep. I have no rest."

Can this state of heightened sensitivity and all-consuming lust be sustained in marriage?

In Song of Songs the couple are never described as being married. It seems, rather, that they are illicit yet ultimately platonic lovers. Their relationship involves neither consummation nor consecration. From here we derive that Eros embodies the twin qualities of hunger (unavailability) and sin.

One of the reasons that marriage sometimes becomes so boring is that it is so legal. Sex is allowed and expected, even obligatory. The thrill of Eros is predicated on the idea of being carried away by something so powerful that we cannot deny or suppress it. It is the pleasure of losing control and being overpowered by something greater than ourselves. Anyone who has ever experienced a truly erotic moment knows what it is to be totally consumed by emotion. It is for this reason – and this is key – that Eros is associated with sin. The force of Eros is such that in its grip you may begin to do things that you are not meant to do. You betray your own principles. You cannot stop yourself from entering the danger zone. You allow yourself to be washed away on a wave of pleasure even as you are dashed against the rocks.

Isn't this the problem with modern life – its boredom and monotony? Nothing carries us away. We have to pull ourselves through the day, as if our lives were some heavy weight attached to our backs and we its beasts of burden. We get up every morning, pulling ourselves out of bed, and then drive our drowsy selves to work. After ten hours in the office, we carry ourselves home, make dinner, do some homework with the kids, and then plunk ourselves down in front of the TV to escape a monotonous existence with scant opportunity for discovery. Nothing makes us feel alive. Future possibility seldom beckons. Soon, we've become old and lethargic and our lives have passed us by.

It's all too predictable. It's all too planned. In essence, we exchange agitation for comfort, danger for safety, anxiety for settled companionship. Yet when there is too much adventure and unpredictability – like there was for some in the generation of the sixties that threw off the rules – there is chaos and anarchy. We don't know how to balance stability and excitement; we always seem to live on one or the other extreme.

How can marriage, predicated as it is on the exclusivity of a contract, ever enjoy the pleasures of sin and Eros? The answer is that life in general, and marriage in particular, must be made sinful. There has to be, strange as it sounds, a sinful and forbidden bedrock within marriage, an illicit contract generating an erotic spark.

By recapturing the erotic we regain the desire to know. Plunging into the mystery of existence, we live everyday life as a totally novel experience. Eroticism transforms life from a destination into a journey, from a passage into an adventure. The Song of Solomon tells us a magical story of a man and a woman who have but one desire: to know each other. But even as they slowly meet in the erotic encounter, they are surrounded by a dark fog of all-encompassing mystery, the second principle of lust. With each interaction they come to know that what there is to know about each other can never be fully known.

The Song's man and woman are mortal lovers who hunger for each other (unavailability), plumb each other's depths (mystery), and share an illicit spark (sinfulness). They also represent God and man, locked in a cosmic relationship, destined to spend an eternity drawing ever closer in love, understanding, and wisdom. In its erotic book, the Bible tempts us to explore the enigma of God, the secrets of the creation, the depths of our own infinite souls: in short, to live a vibrant life of Eros.

Devekut – Cleaving

Passion and vibrancy are hardwired into creation. Isn't this what God demonstrates to His people – a deep yearning? And it's what God wants us to have for Him as well. The Bible enjoins us to cleave to God, to bind with Him in what is called in Hebrew *devekut*, meaning the state of cleaving or clinging, from the root *devek* (spelled with the Hebrew letters *daled, bet, kuf*), meaning glue:

> After the Lord your God shall ye walk, and Him shall ye fear, and His commandments shall ye keep, and unto His voice shall ye hearken, and Him shall ye serve, and unto Him shall ye cleave [*u'bo tidbakun*].[83]

This is precisely the same language used in the Bible's instruction for a man and wife to cleave together:

> Therefore shall a man leave his father and his mother, and shall cleave unto his wife [*v'davak b'ishto*], and they shall be one flesh. (Genesis 2:24)[84]

Isn't that the whole problem with religion – that we don't covet God enough? That we are very complacent in our spiritual relationship? That ritual can be bereft of passion? We engage in religious obligations, but there's no real desire; there's no real lust. We may love God but it's kind of boring. And it doesn't invigorate us. It doesn't make us feel passionate about God. This is why so many people today embrace various forms of mysticism – they are yearning for an intensity of spiritual connection.

Jewish literature is replete with references to a lusty and passionate relationship with God. Take the famous poem "Yedid Nefesh" (beloved of the soul), thought to have been written by the sixteenth-century kabbalist Rabbi Elazar ben Moshe Azikri. Sung on various occasions in Jewish liturgy (including notably the beginning of the Sabbath as well as at that day's third meal, and by many Chassidim daily before beginning the morning prayers), the poem speaks of a deep yearning for God: *Ki zeh kamah nichsof nichsafti...*, "How much have I pined for you, O God." *Nichsof nichsafti* comes from the root word *kosef* (spelled with the Hebrew letters *kaf, samech, feh*), meaning yearning, longing, or deep desire, and related to the word *kesef*, meaning silver or money – things universally wanted.

Some eight hundred years ago the twelfth-century sage Abraham ibn Ezra composed his beautiful song "Tzama

Nafshi," sung by many Jews at the Sabbath meal on Friday nights, to express his soul's yearning for the Creator: *Tzama nafshi l'Elokim l'Kel chai*, "My soul thirsts for God, for the living God," *libi u'vesari yeranenu l'Kel chai*, "my heart and my flesh will sing to the living God."

God wants to be desired by us, and likewise our souls yearn for God in a mutual intense bond. God is not cold or complacent or detached. He is involved rather than aloof, immersed rather than indifferent. God is discovered not in the monotony of subsistence but in the ecstasy of living. But today we have rejected the God of wonder and replaced Him with the God of cheap tricks, a God that serves for many as a furry rabbit's foot, a form of superstition. If Nietzsche was right and God is dead, then that can only be because man has killed Him off. We don't pray because we have a flame burning in our hearts, but because we have debts burning in our pockets. Our prayers are shallow attempts at deal making, cynical business transactions: *God, You do for me, and I'll do for You.*

If we are not passionate in our spiritual relationships, we won't be in our physical relationships either. Eros is an all-encompassing way of viewing the world. The Song of Solomon challenges us to feel for God and life what a man and a woman feel for each other in the heat of passion. The Song challenges us to be erotically charged in our religious commitments. For a man who tries to uncover the mysteries of a beautiful woman, every interaction is emotionally pointed. He pursues her not because he wants something from her but because she excites him. Even if he never tastes of her sensual pleasures but merely beholds her from a distance, in awe and wonder, he is still enraptured. God wants to be the people's mistress. He wants to be exciting to us for His very existence, not because He can bless us to win the lottery.

God wants us to thrill to the study of His law, delight in the fulfillment of His commandments, revel in uncovering the mysteries of the universe, and soar in fathoming the mysteries of His name. It is no coincidence that Kabbalah employs extensive sexual imagery in depicting the relationship between God and man. The sexual instinct is all consuming, and the saintly righteous are obsessed with God's existence. Theirs is a form of spiritual yearning and hunger that is utterly undeniable and irrepressible.

This is why study is so central to the Jewish faith. At its core Eros is a manifestation of a desire to know. Eroticism's heart and soul is curiosity. To be erotically attracted to a woman is to want to know every fiber of her heart and every inch of her person. To live without Eros is to fundamentally lose a desire to appreciate and apprehend. The three rules of Eros are to be found in Song of Songs. By unlocking Eros, the Song serves as the soul of the Bible, the spirit within God's word, all of which is about life and its secrets.

> It is no coincidence that Kabbalah employs extensive sexual imagery in depicting the relationship between God and man. The sexual instinct is all consuming, and the saintly righteous are obsessed with God's existence.

I counseled a married man who said he had an affair because, unlike his wife, his mistress made him feel like he was more than a provider. To his wife he had felt that the only thing that mattered was that he was a breadwinner, a reliable partner and parent. But the other woman tried to take away his pain. She wanted to know his heart rather than his hands.

She made him feel human again, he said. "I want to know the things that worry you, that disappoint you. Your hurts, your pain. I want to know whether you feel like you're a success or a failure. I want to be a comfort to you." This man's wife, he said, had never spoken to him in those terms. She loved him, but she didn't want to *know* him.

Now, we can dismiss his words as the rationalizations and excuses of a man seeking to justify his immoral action and, indeed, there is no excuse for adultery. It is a horrible sin that causes unimaginable pain. But I encounter many a husband who feels that he is appreciated for what he produces rather than what he is.

The same, of course, is true of women. Every woman is, to borrow a phrase from Winston Churchill, "a riddle, wrapped in a mystery, inside an enigma." And every secret seeks to be revealed, just as every dark night is ultimately abolished by the rays of the morning sun. A woman wants a man to know her secret. It is not principally her clothes she wants removed but rather her layers stripped away. And while most men are fine at the former, the overwhelming majority, especially husbands, are terrible at the latter.

To live without Eros – to subsist in ignorance without the desire to know deeply – is a life of darkness. It is a wretched existence. To live with *devekut*, cleaving to God and to one's spouse, is a life of passion, excitement, and vibrancy. That is a life worth living.

Biblical Marriages

Marriages can be broken into two types: the friendship marriage and the lust marriage. While you might expect that the Bible would advocate a marriage of collegial friendship or a model of quiet and calm love, marriages that are discussed in the Torah are really much more about lust than about love and friendship. *Ma'aseh avos siman l'banim*, "what happens to the fathers is an omen for the children," says the Midrash Tanchuma, quoted by the Jewish sage Nachmanides in his commentary on Genesis 12:6. The three patriarchs – Abraham, Isaac, and Jacob – are the forerunners of the Jewish people. Whatever happens to them becomes the model for Jewish history, so it is instructive to look at what the Bible says about their marriages. The example of all three patriarchs' marriages shows that the archetypal biblical marriage in the Five Books of Moses is one built on fiery passion.

ABRAHAM AND SARAH

The "friendship marriage" is built on love and familiarity. Abraham and Sarah don't have that. This is the type of relationship where a man says, "My wife is my best friend." I've never really understood that expression. I've always seen it as a little bit of an insult. She's your best friend – what do you guys do? Watch the football game together? Eat Doritos with salsa? Do you *belch* together? You mean you're not lovers but you just kind of dorm together? If you think about it, "best friend" connotes a very familiar relationship that's not based on deep desire. And I'll prove it: you don't marry your best friend. You share an apartment with him or her and talk about your girlfriends or boyfriends.

This is not to say that a married couple should not be friends. Friendship is absolutely an essential and fundamental dimension to every happy marriage. You have to feel comfortable with each other, make each other laugh, and comfort one another. But if a husband and wife relate to each other primarily as friends, they are missing a critical aspect of the potential relationship they are meant to have. In essence, husband and wife being best friends is, at best, half a relationship. The other, more important half is being lovers.

The "lust marriage," in contrast to the cozy familiarity of the "friendship marriage," is based on distance. The lust we're talking about is what Abraham felt for Sarah. You'll notice that Abraham says to Sarah as they're going down to Egypt, *I need you to tell a white lie, dear, that we're brother and sister, because if Pharaoh knows that I'm your husband he'll kill me.* And Abraham says to Sarah, *hinei na yadati ki ishah yefat mareh at*, "behold, I now know that you're a beautiful woman (Genesis 12:11)." Most translations join the word *na* (now) to *hinei* (behold), rendering "Behold now, I know that you're a beautiful woman."[85] But others translate according to a comment made by the canonical commentator Rashi, who reads, according to the Midrash, "Behold, I now know that you are a beautiful woman." Abraham and Sarah had been married for decades. I *now* know that you're a beautiful woman? And why didn't he know before?

The Midrash, as Rashi explains, indicates that until now Abraham did not know that Sarah was beautiful because they practiced distance in their relationship even though they'd been married for decades. They were careful never to let their marriage suffer from overfamiliarity. Only now, chancing to see Sarah's reflection in the Nile as they travel, does Abraham realize how comely is his wife.[86] They have maintained mystery and even obstacles between them rather than the kind of familiarity that can breed love but also predictability and contempt. This kind of distance is an example of "the erotic obstacle." Only with obstacles to total familiarity can a couple maintain erotic interest. This is the modern secret that our forefather and foremother Abraham and Sarah understood more than 3,700 years ago.

Abraham and Sarah did not spend every waking hour together; they maintained some separateness. We see this in Genesis when Abraham is receiving three mysterious visitors: "'Where is your wife Sarah?' they asked him. 'There, in the tent,' he said" (Genesis 8:9). Rashi explains that Abraham is extolling his wife's virtue: she is modest and does not parade herself in front of male guests. But furthermore, she is maintaining her own quarters and her own separate activities. She has her domain and he has his.

A couple that maintains separate interests and activities has more to bring to each other when they do come together. The separateness enhances the togetherness. Abraham and Sarah had a joint spiritual mission – to spread monotheism and knowledge of the One God throughout the world. Yet each of them brought separate strengths to their common goal and they worked in parallel but not without independence. When the two of them left their former home of Haran, at God's direction, to go to the land that would later be known as the Land of Israel, the Bible tells us that they took with them *hanefesh asher asu*, "the souls that they had made" (Genesis 12:5).[87] Rashi comments that these were people whom Abraham and Sarah had taught spiritually, and he feels the need to specify that *Avraham megayer et ha'anashim v'Sarah*

> Only with obstacles to total familiarity can a couple maintain erotic interest. This is the modern secret that our forefather and foremother Abraham and Sarah understood more than 3,700 years ago.

megayeret hanashim, "Abraham converted the men and Sarah converted the women." Each had a separate task to perform. The two of them were spiritually conjoined in the deepest possible way – but without being joined at the hip.

ISAAC AND REBECCA

The first time they met, as Rebecca approached on a camel and saw her husband-to-be from afar, Rebecca "took her veil and covered herself" (Genesis 24:65). She made sure she was never totally known by her husband; her very first action in their relationship was to create unavailability and mystery. Apparently it worked: we know that the couple had a positive lustful relationship, based on Genesis 26:8: *Yitzchak metzachek et Rivka ishto,* "Isaac was jesting with his wife Rebecca."[88] Rashi infers that this refers to sexual playfulness and indicates Isaac and Rebecca were engaged in marital relations.[89]

Note that this incident of playful relations took place more than thirty-five years after Isaac and Rebecca married (they married when Isaac was 40 [Genesis 25:20; Rebecca's age is not specified in the Bible]; their twins Jacob and Esau were born when Isaac was 60 [Genesis 25:26]; and this incident follows the one in which Esau sold his birthright for a bowl of lentils [Genesis 25:29–34], said to have occurred when the twins were fifteen years old[90]). Isaac was presumably over seventy-five years old, then, when he intimately "jested" or "sported" with his wife, so we can infer that the lustful dimension between the two of them must have been quite strong to have remained so joyful after so many years together!

JACOB AND RACHEL

No discussion of lust in biblical marriages would be complete without an intensive look at the relationship between Jacob and Rachel. When Jacob first sees Rachel, he is overcome. His immediate reaction is to help her by rolling away a large stone from the mouth of the well where she has come to water her father's sheep (Genesis 29:10). This was clearly no mean feat; it was a task normally accomplished by a whole group of men (Genesis 29:3), yet Jacob was immediately able to roll the giant stone off the well by himself after having gotten a glimpse of Rachel.

From the first instant Jacob's desire for Rachel was incredibly strong and real. He could not suppress it. This was not love. It was hunger, lust: deep, unquenchable desire. It's what we would call immediate chemistry. But make no mistake: this was not just a physical reaction. It was the yearning of two souls who had been predestined for one another.

After having watered the sheep for Rachel, "Jacob kissed Rachel and began to weep aloud" (Genesis 29:11). The kissing is obvious, but why did he weep? Rashi explains that Jacob wept upon foreseeing that he and Rachel would not be buried together.[91] Lust is magnified through erotic obstacles and loss: this is the first rule of lust, unavailability. Jacob cries when he envisions that he can never fully possess Rachel. Their life together will be cut short. Rachel will tragically die in childbirth as their second son together is born, and she will be buried on the road to Bethlehem as they travel (Genesis 35:18–19). Jacob will eventually be buried with Leah (Genesis 49:31, 50:13), not Rachel; he will not share his eternal rest with this woman for whom his soul pines.

In this initial scene of their meeting, it is clear that Jacob immediately saw Rachel as his intended from the moment he laid eyes on her, and also that he was bowled over by the intensity of his feelings. Yet can it be said that he loved her at this point? He didn't even know her! Jacob's immediate feelings for Rachel are the yearning of one soul for another, the magnetic gravitation of two spiritual energies. This was a tremendously powerful desire, a force so irresistible that Jacob was willing to pay almost any price. He forthwith announces to her father Laban, "I'll work for you seven years in return for your younger daughter Rachel" (Genesis 29:18).

Now listen to this: it's one of the most romantic verses contained in any literature, not just the Bible. *Va'yihyu b'einav k'yamim echadim b'ahavato otah*, "it appeared in his eyes as if it were but days, so much did he long for her" (Genesis 29:20).[92] And the Bible here uses the phrase *b'ahavato otah*, "in his love for her." But this emotion, this longing, is not the familiar, cozy kind of love that we extol today in Western society. Obviously the word *love* here means something stronger. It refers to the kind of deep longing and lust that has a man pine so deeply for a woman that it transports him above time and space. You have to desire someone *immensely* to lose total track of time as Jacob did.

Indeed, what did Jacob say at the end of the seven years? "Give me my wife. My time is completed, and I want to make love to her" (Genesis 29:21). Due to Laban's duplicity, Jacob would in fact have to work another seven years for Rachel, but that's another story, and the fact that he did so testifies to the continued strength of his longing and of the force of the bond of lust that drew the patriarch to his favored wife.

PART 3

Sinfulness: Getting to Forbidden Territory

Chapter 7

Vive la Différence: Magnetizing Marriage

Keep Your Distance

The Jewish marriage's foundation in lust – and not love – is plainly visible in Jewish law: the three principles of lust – unavailability, mystery, and forbiddenness – are all introduced into the Jewish marriage by Jewish law. Not only do we see from this that lust in the long term is possible, but also that Jewish law considers it to be fundamental.

The quality of unavailability is readily evident in Jewish law, and is seen to a high degree in traditional Jewish communities even today. Men and women sit separately in the synagogue and at celebrations and are largely educated in unisex institutions.

The classically understood reason why religious Jewish men and women keep their distance is to keep people from being compromised. It doesn't take too much imagination to envision the kind of problems people can get into when the boundaries between men and women are too fluid. Take David Petraeus. He's a great American hero, and we're all in his debt. He saved America from humiliation in the Iraq war, he helped save many Arab lives, and he made sure that a lot of bad guys were eliminated. But he went jogging with a doting young woman and got a little bit too close. Judaism says you have to be careful there – Jewish law forbids men and women who aren't married from being behind closed doors together alone. Being too private with a woman who's not your wife can lead to very sticky situations.

But that's not the only reason. The other reason is precisely the opposite: not that you could grow too intimate, but that you could grow too familiar and become inured to the natural attraction that is supposed to develop between men and women. There has to be a little bit of distance. When there's a little bit of distance, a little bit of unavailability, it actually fosters attraction.

Traditional Jews do not believe in coeducation. I know that this debate continues to be a heated one around America. What we usually focus on in the debate about coed versus single-sex education is the question of what makes a better educational environment for boys and girls. A lot of women and a lot of female educators feel that single-sex classrooms are a better environment for women, and the studies show that girls in particular excel in single-sex education.[93] Why should young women have to be self-conscious about things like appearance and popularity in their formative years when they're supposed to be focused on education?

But that's a different conversation. No one seems to focus on whether it's healthy for the kind of affectionate bonds that are supposed to naturally grow between boys and girls to have that level of familiarity from such an early age. Gender difference can be slowly eroded through overexposure. Boys and girls sit in class together, play together, grow up together, learn sex-ed together. They even wear the same clothes. There's not a whole lot of barriers separating them, and most young Americans have platonic friends of both sexes. Hanging out with members of the opposite sex is no big deal. By the time you get to a secular university campus, so much of the magic and the mystery has already worn off, as Allan Bloom says so poignantly in *The Closing of the American Mind*, based on what he saw for thirty years at institutions like Yale, Cornell, and the University of Chicago. "On reflection," he notes, "today's students wonder what all the fuss was about."[94]

We've created a society where all polarity has been erased from the relationship between men and women. There's no unavailability – men and women are exposed to each other from the earliest age. The problem is not so much that sex has been degraded through a culture of permissiveness, but rather that it has lost its potency through a culture of homogeneity and overexposure. Sex has become banal; it no longer has transformative power.

> The problem is not so much that sex has been degraded through a culture of permissiveness, but rather that it has lost its potency through a culture of homogeneity and overexposure. Sex has become banal; it no longer has transformative power.

This is why the Jewish religion insists on keeping distance between men and women. Even in external appearance, men and women are supposed to be separate. The Bible mandates certain incontrovertible differences that must forever remain between men and women. It says that men cannot wear women's clothing (Deuteronomy 22:5) and men are not to uproot the hair on their faces (Leviticus 19:27; this is why I sport my super-sexy Abraham Lincoln mountain-man beard look). Men are meant to look like men, and women are meant to look like women. Of course, men today shave and women wear pants. But beyond the requirements of religious law and my own commitment to the dictates of the Bible, the larger point is that how we dress should capture a certain masculine or feminine presence, respectively, that increases attraction and draws the sexes toward one another.

But in Western society today, men and women look increasingly homogenous. Pick up any copy of *Vogue* or *Cosmopolitan* from the last fifty years and you can't help but notice how mainstream the masculinization of the female body has become. Starting with Twiggy in the 1960s, the most prestigious models are the ones who look more like pre-teen boys than women – or even girls. They have no body fat, no breasts, nor even hips. But while it all appears harmless, becoming a unisex society is something we should seek to avoid if we don't want to be demagnetized to the opposite sex. And the more we accent gender difference, the greater the attraction will be.

A man I know became traditionally religious after having grown up secular. Once an old friend of his came to visit him in his religious neighborhood. When the secular friend got closer to the religious man's house, he called on his cell phone to ask for directions. As he drove through the streets of what was for him an exotic locale, he suddenly exclaimed, "Man, religious women are hot!" Keep in mind these women were covered up from just under their chins to below the elbows and knees!

I've always seen the intense kind of attraction that secular men have for religiously attired women, because they're used to women who have been slightly masculinized, so when they're hit with the sexual polarity of a truly feminine woman, they're blown away. That's why people like period movies of Jane Austen novels. Why would men want to see women in eighteenth-century clothing? Don't men just want to see women in bikinis? It turns out that what they really want is to see women dressed in ways totally different from men: they're craving the sexual polarity that has been all but neutralized in our society.

Adam and Eve had perfect polarity because he was Man and she was Woman. There was only one woman in the whole world, and Adam was therefore attracted to womankind. Today, that polarity has been diluted and instead of man being attracted to womankind, man is attracted only to a certain *kind* of woman. The effect of homogeneity, overexposure of the sexes to each other from a young age, and the consequent dilution of sexual polarity is that men are not attracted in a blanket way to femininity. A woman? Who cares, no big deal! In our unisex culture, there is so little to differentiate men and women from each other. To attract male attention today, it's not enough for a woman to be a woman; she almost has to be exceptionally beautiful.

Besides, in today's casual "hookup" culture, sex is so readily and easily available. There's nothing special about it. It's calculated, arranged for convenience and with minimal commitment, as described by "A," a junior at the University of Pennsylvania interviewed for a *New York Times* article on the hookup culture on campus: "We [women on campus] are very aware of cost-benefit issues and trading up and trading down, so no one wants to be too tied to someone that, you know, may not be the person they want to be with in a couple of months."[95] Hookups are about a purely physical encounter that is casual in the extreme and comes without the commitment of a relationship ("We don't really like each other in person, sober," noted the Penn junior about her hookup partner[96]).

Beyond that, people are utterly overexposed to sexuality through the constant bombardment of sexual imagery and discussion in the media. If you live in America and you have turned on your radio or TV, walked down the street, gone into a mall, or opened a magazine or newspaper, chances are you have been looking at sexually charged images or provocatively dressed people. The sight becomes "ho hum." To get your interest it's going to have to be something really outstanding.

Most men in America are attracted to perhaps 20 percent of the female population. The same (rather masculinized, incidentally) female form is offered to us in all the magazines and movies, conforming to a stereotyped ideal, like the blonde Nordic type typical of Tiger Woods' mistresses.

But let me ask you this: If the definition of a heterosexual male is someone who's attracted to women, and we're only attracted to something like a fifth of the female population, are we still heterosexual? Our manhood, our masculinity, has been compromised!

And it's painful for women, as well, because they have to adapt to that stereotype of what the culture will determine is attractive at any given time. Every woman wants to look like that no more than a fifth of the female population that's considered ideal. Women today are made to feel like they're never blond enough, never blue-eyed enough, their legs are never long enough, their chests are never large enough, and for sure they're never young enough or thin enough. That's the cultural standard of beauty, so women look in the mirror and always see something that's kind of ugly to them, thereby forgetting what all studies show – that the sexiest quality of all is self-confidence. When you carry yourself confidently, people are drawn to you, but when you carry yourself with self-loathing, you begin to lose your natural magnetism.

When I talk about sexual polarity, however, I'm not just talking about appearances. I'm talking about masculine and feminine energies. Not just the stereotypical qualities associated with men and women, but the primal, core energies each sex possesses.

Men are naturally pursuers. Their very biology suggests an outward reach. And I believe women want to be the ones who are pursued. I'm not saying women can't pursue men – they can. But it can't be the essence of the relationship, and it has to be done in a feminine manner. Where women lose their dignity in pursuing a man, the man feels he's almost being stalked. Yes, it may be a double standard and unfair. But it's a reality nonetheless. In their heart of hearts, men want to be the ones who do the pursuing and women want to be the ones who are pursued. Feminine energy on the other hand is naturally nurturing. The gravitation of the masculine to the feminine is met with the response of the nurturing of the masculine by the feminine.

For the record, I am a feminist (and a father of six very competent daughters). I believe women can do everything men do, but *they can do so as women*. My wife can do anything that I can do, and she works with me in all my projects, but she does things very differently from me. There's a ladylike quality to her; you see it in her smile, in the way she knows how to create a hospitable atmosphere in the home, something our many guests immediately notice. She also experiences life in a far more sensitive and deeply emotionally connected way than I do. I envy that connection, and I think it's something to be celebrated.

In our aggressive world, we tend to look at that kind of emotional connectivity and sensitivity as weakness. Instead we should be celebrating the differences between the natural male and female energies, and men should be learning from their wives how to be more emotionally available. Think about it: God is the master of the universe. He could have made us unisex. But he didn't: "male and female He created them" (Genesis 1:27).

Gary suffered a major trauma when his sister was killed in a car accident. He withdrew into a very dark period. Unfortunately, he took it out on his wife, Cheryl. Gary began to criticize Cheryl constantly. Everything she did was wrong. If she bought him a shirt, it was the wrong size or too expensive; if she cooked dinner, it wasn't what he liked, and so on. In the face of Gary's harshness, Cheryl just went sour on him. Instead of trying to talk to him about what was happening to him, she distanced herself emotionally. When Gary resisted her early attempts to be nurturing, Cheryl adopted a very masculine mode in turn. She went cold, barely spoke to Gary, gave him monosyllabic answers, and so on.

By the time I spoke to Gary and Cheryl they were hardly speaking to each other. Cheryl told me, "If he was warm to me, I would try, but he's so cold, I can't do it." I urged her to make an effort to reach out to her husband, who had suffered a terrible tragedy, but her response was, "I'm sorry, I didn't make the tragedy. I tried to be comforting but he rejects it and pushes me away." I suggested to Cheryl that Gary was testing her. "He doesn't feel loved right now," I told her. "He feels isolated and alone, and he's pushing you away in the hope that you're going to say 'I'm never going to abandon you.' But when you respond coldly to him, he says to himself, 'See, she doesn't love me. Nobody loves me.'"

In fact Gary was in the grips of powerful feelings of guilt over his sister's death. Of course the accident had not been his fault, but because he had suggested to his sister that she go to a certain place, he felt responsible. Gary felt very isolated, very abandoned. No one understood what he was experiencing. I tried to get Cheryl to see it from his point of view. "You're kind of proving to him that he was correct all along that he's not loved," I challenged her, "that you'll only love him under certain circumstances."

Cheryl took my words to heart and started trying to make some overtures to her husband, but Gary confided to me that he no longer wanted to be intimate with his wife. "Because she was cold to you, you're going to punish her?" I asked him. He said, "No, I'm really not attracted to her. She was so aggressive, so mean." I pointed out that Gary had been aggressive and mean to Cheryl as well. "That's the whole point," he said." If we're both like that then how can we have any kind of relationship?"

The polarity in this relationship had been lost. He was angry, she was angry. They were both in an aggressive masculine mode, and there was no feminine pole in the relationship. Without polarity, there was no spark of connection.

Sometimes sex has the power to overcome hurt and pain. In my book *Kosher Sex* I actually advocated that couples could use sex to help solve problems. I was roundly criticized for that, but I stand by the point: it's not that you should use sex to paper over problems, but to take some of the sting out of the fighting so that you can actually talk. Men are so drawn to a nurturing feminine presence, and women are so drawn to a strong, protecting masculine presence. Sometimes you have to tap into the power of sex to overcome hurt feelings. But this power comes from the polarity of the relationship: when there is no polarity, the sexual relationship loses its power.

For a married couple, maintaining some separateness in your lives is a healthy way to promote the delicious difference that keeps attraction alive and vibrant. A couple do not have to do everything together. They can also have independent friends and activities. It is good for the relationship to do your separate things sometimes and not always be joined at the hip. Being apart at times only makes it more explosive when you come back together.

And don't be afraid to embrace your natural core energies. Men: feel free to pursue your wives. Stare at your wife the way you once did. Call her from work to tell her that you're calling for no other reason than you were thinking about her. Treat her like she is single and you are still wooing her. Chances are she is waiting to be chased. Women: feel free to nurture your husbands. Offering a listening ear for his worries is a caring gesture that will likely be repaid double in his attention to you. Your kindness is a balm for his soul.

Curb TMI

A popular acronym these days is "TMI" – too much information. This is used to describe the squirmy feeling you get when someone has divulged way more than you ever wanted to know, leaving absolutely no mystery. Unfortunately, a lot of marriages are suffering from such overexposure. There is a good reason that Jewish values dictate that a wife should preserve a modicum of modesty even in the bedroom and that a husband should be careful never to attend to his hygienic needs in his wife's presence. Not everything in marriage is designed to be shared. I've counseled many married couples and it's fascinating to me how people think that marriage is license to parade around the bedroom completely naked all the time, without people realizing that that's exactly how the human body loses its magnetism. The most boring place to ever visit is a nudist colony. (Er... or so my friends tell me.)

What's sexier, a short skirt, or a long skirt with a slit? A nude woman, or a woman in a long gown that suggests the form of her body or has translucent lace sections? "Peekaboo" is always more enticing than "let it all hang out." Am I right? This is because of the inherent sexiness of mystery.

> There is a good reason that Jewish values dictate that a wife should preserve a modicum of modesty even in the bedroom and that a husband should be careful never to attend to his hygienic needs in his wife's presence. Not everything in marriage is designed to be shared.

Daniel and Kelly were alienated from each other and were having sex only about once a month when they came to see me. Kelly told me she was desperate for her husband to notice her, and had even told him that if things didn't change, she was at risk of having an affair. Kelly was a very open type. She often walked around the house wearing very little clothing – even in front of the kids. Yet not only was Daniel not responding to her, he was even harsh: "You don't know how to be sexy," he told Kelly. "You just don't know how to be a woman."

One day out of the blue Daniel told Kelly he wanted her to wear stockings – and only stockings – while they had sex. Kelly was hesitant. It wasn't her style. "That's kind of weird," she said to me in counseling, "don't you think? Why would he want that?" I said first of all, who cares why he wants it? When one spouse is expressing a fantasy, it's an opportunity to increase intimacy and I recommend that spouses try to be accommodating whenever possible. But beyond that, I told Kelly that it seemed pretty obvious to me that Daniel simply wanted to see her more covered up, more mysterious. Kelly was an open book – there wasn't anything mysterious about her, and Daniel just couldn't get interested. He needed her to be more concealed; this was the ingredient that had been missing for him to find her sexy. Kelly wore the stockings, and Daniel's interest was rekindled.

The most important holy relics in the Jewish faith are always concealed. When you walk into a synagogue, interestingly, the holiest object – the Torah scroll – is nowhere to be seen. It's hidden behind a *parochet* (a heavy curtain that covers the ark), behind the wooden doors of the ark (a sort of cupboard), and underneath a heavy cloth mantle. We revere it. When it finally makes an appearance, brought forth from the ark, we stand up for it. We are careful what we say in its presence. If it falls, God forbid, we fast for forty days – something holy has been violated. Are we bringing any of this kind of reverence into our marriages? Is the holy covenant of marriage sacred for us? Is our relationship precious and valuable? Do we protect it with a veil of privacy and mystery?

I see married couples who give friends the house tour, and they take them all around the house – "this is the kitchen, this is the living room, here's our bedroom" – as if the place where a couple makes love is just like any other room in the house. It's a public space. There's no sacredness associated with it, nothing unavailable or mysterious. It's just part of the house tour! If so, then you've made your bedroom into a public space. It's tantamount to saying that nothing uniquely intimate takes place there, instead of maintaining the sanctity of your intimate relationship.

The same thing is true, by the way, when it comes to having children in the bedroom on a regular basis, which is not healthy for children, and it's not healthy for a marriage. Appropriate boundaries should be observed.

Eroticism flourishes in an atmosphere of mystery and hiddenness. Modesty enhances the erotic quality of the human body and imposes erotic barriers that must be overcome in order to obtain the object of desire. When there are no obstacles, there is no mystery and no power to the intensity of the intimate experience. This is ancient wisdom. Legend has it that a few hundred years ago a young woman wrote to a Jewish sage with a dilemma. She was raised to be modest her whole life, she told him, totally separate from men – never even talked to them. How then, she wanted to know, could she be expected to contradict her upbringing and go the total opposite extreme on her wedding night of experiencing full-out sexual intimacy, on the very first night she really knew a man? The sage answered her that this is not a contradiction. The whole reason you've preserved your modesty until now, he advised her, is to enhance the power of that night.

Jason, a very romantic young man whose parents were divorced, was seventeen years old when he had his first sexual experience. Or he would have had his first sexual experience, if he hadn't walked out. He had gotten to know a girl and they were becoming friends. One night they were sitting around in her bedroom talking about music, and all of a sudden she just took off her blouse and her bra. Totally taken aback, Jason mumbled an excuse about having to be somewhere and he left. It wasn't that she wasn't pretty, he told me, or that he was intimidated, either. He just couldn't believe that his first experience would be so casual, so devoid of mystery, so ordinary. He had thought the first time would be magical, not just a random moment utterly without prelude.

This is why pornography is in fact not at all erotic. The more you examine real eroticism, the more you realize that porn lacks all three of its components. Pornography is not at all unavailable, especially in the Internet age. It is not mysterious – there is no modesty or hiddenness involved whatsoever. And furthermore, it isn't sinful: What could be less forbidden than legally paying someone to pose for naked photographs? The models have all signed legal consent forms! Beyond that, porn has an inherent contradiction in it. The essence of eroticism and the reason why it's so powerful is that it celebrates our ability to surrender ourselves to a mysterious force beyond ourselves. Is there anything more unnatural or downright silly than people *acting as if* that power is overwhelming them? Faking it? That's why porn is ultimately so boring and unsatisfying.

Why be satisfied with a mockery when we could delve into true mystery? The human soul longs for depth and enigma. Space has such a deep hold on our imagination because it is limitless and unknown. People used to have that kind of hunger for God. Nowadays we like to put everything in a box. Americans love lists: every year we have the top fifty this and the ten best that. People want to quantify, objectify, remove all curiosity. Real lust actually is not about objectifying. It's about stripping away the external and getting to the core energy, where the masculine wants to gravitate towards the feminine, the feminine wants to nurture the masculine, and the energy is limitless.

Get into Mischief

We've seen that the very legality of marriage tends to work against lust, since it contradicts the third principle of erotic attraction. It's a quandary: How can a marriage be sinful? Isn't the whole reason you got married so that the relationship is now legal, so you're no longer living in sin? And yet, a married couple in Judaism live in sin for twelve days out of every month. The forbidden and sinful is incorporated into the marital state. Based on several biblical passages (Leviticus 15:19 and 24, 18:19, and 20:18), Jewish law specifies the parameters of the intimate marital relationship: for approximately twelve days out of every month – the days of menstruation and seven days thereafter – a man's wife becomes forbidden to him. Not only may he not have sex with her, he also may not share her bed, kiss her, or hug her. In fact, he is completely forbidden to touch her. The relationship becomes illicit. Suddenly, from the confines of the routine and the predictable emerges the sinful and the erotic. And because he may not consummate his lust, he learns to hunger without end.

When a man can see everything, he chooses not to see. Because he has seen it all. Because there is nothing new. Until he is not allowed to see, not supposed to see. And now, does he ever want to see! It is specifically in the resistance created by erotic obstacles and barriers that passion is to be found. This is why Jewish law has the wisdom to suddenly disallow sex after about half a month. After the two weeks together, the three conditions of lust begin to disappear: it's too legal, too available, and lust begins to dissipate. We can learn from this the importance of never allowing the three principles of lust to go untended. We must constantly strive to introduce and reintroduce the elements of unavailability, mystery, and sinfulness into our marriages.

Keep the ultimate goal in mind, however: the sinfulness has to be within bounds. An affair is the ultimate sinfulness. It's definitely erotic. It's also incredibly destructive. Bringing a third party into your marriage bears a terrible cost. Eroticism is a fire. You have to have a fire in your house or your house will be freezing cold – you won't be able to live in it. But the fire has to be maintained and it has to be guarded in a fireplace. You can't let the fire burn in the kitchen – the whole house will go up. That's why these things have to be contained in their proper boundaries. So how do you bring some forbiddenness into the relationship without getting into destructive territory? How do you make your spouse off limits in a healthy way that fans the flames where you want them fanned?

We can learn something from a concept in Jewish law that involves separating things into their component parts. For example, the Fifth Commandment enjoins us to honor our parents. What if you have a surrogate mother? To whom do you owe this honor: to the biological mother, or the one who raised you? What is the critical part of being a mother?

We can extend this concept of breaking things into their component parts to an analysis of ways to increase erotic attraction by bringing the forbidden into our marriages. Take the example of an affair. I argued in my book *Kosher Adultery* for having an affair with your spouse. There are many suggestions in that book for bringing the illicit into your life in productive ways and turning your marriage into a steamy affair.

Let's try to separate out the elements of another erotic game: courtly love.

Back in the twelfth century, in the days of Eleanor of Aquitaine, the mother of Richard the Lionheart, there was an interesting practice that bears modern scrutiny. In those misty royal environs, courtly love is said to have been born. This is how it worked: A knight would choose a woman, usually married, to whom he would pay homage. He would do everything to win the hand of the unwinnable matron. She was more often than not wedded to a nobleman far above the knight's station. As a social and financial inferior, he had little chance of ever winning over the hand of the fair, not to mention married, maiden. Leaving her husband for someone far below her status, however gallant, would have been a costly mistake on her part. But that did not mean that the woman in question did not enjoy basking in the adulation of her knight in shining armor. He would do everything to impress her. Before jousting he would request that she allow him to tie her bow to his lance. Before going out to battle he would tell her he was dedicating his sword in her honor and ask her to pray for his safe return. All this was done in the full view and knowledge of husbands, who arguably did not take offense, seeing as they were doing the same with some other unattainable woman who was herself above their social station. So, a duke might be paying homage to his queen, a baron to a duchess, and so on.

What guaranteed the longevity of the man's desire for the woman was specifically her forbiddenness to him. His inability to ever consummate the relationship kept him in a state of deliberate longing. Now, one can imagine that a society filled with people who were always longing for people they were not married to led to a great deal of lust but also a great deal of marital misery. Then there is the simple immorality of married couples allowing others to intrude upon the intimacy of their union.

The fact is, however, that almost every wife does have an admirer, whether she knows it or not. Men cast their eye on women. Even a pious, religious woman may get stared at without her even being aware of it. Most husbands don't realize that other men might be looking at their wives. Since they themselves are not attracted to their own wives, they can't imagine some other guy is attracted to them. And even if he is, they're usually not fazed because they're certainly not threatened by it. Sadly there is not enough jealousy. A man who looks at his wife every night and is so unexcited that he turns to the television set may not think of her as someone who would inspire attraction.

But what if a husband does notice other men's interest in his wife? This may spark an erotic conversation that probes some of the darkness and mystery of attraction. This is just one example of embracing forbiddenness through fantasy. At the very least, a man's awareness of his wife's inherent attractiveness is essential to his own attraction to her.

Let's go further with the idea of courtly admirers and tweak the system slightly. What if husbands themselves were to become their wives' admirers? What if they were to send their wives anonymous notes? Play erotic games? What if you called up your wife in the middle of the day and told her you've booked a hotel room to meet her at?

Fantasy is another tool to uncover some of the hidden layers of the erotic mind. Fantasy is incredibly powerful. Female fantasy is often much more erotic than the male variety (which has a tendency to be pornographic). Part of being married is constant exploration. Sex has a million permutations. It's like chess: you can have an infinite number of moves. I don't just mean physical moves. There are a million questions that can be asked that probe the erotic details of your spouse's mind. After years together, couples begin to think there's nothing left to discover, but if you make an effort to have these kinds of erotic conversations with your spouse, you may be amazed to discover what lies beneath the surface.

I once counseled a couple who were struggling with their sex life. The husband didn't feel attracted to the wife, and things were not going smoothly in the bedroom. One day during our session the wife revealed to her husband that she had a specific sexual fantasy about him. This piqued his interest and he wanted to hear more. This man was raised in Russia and spoke the language fluently, even though his wife did not. "I fantasize about you telling me in Russian all these things that you want me to do to you, and I have to guess what they are because I don't understand what you're saying." This fantasy revealed something very deep in this woman's mind: she wanted to know if the two of them spoke a universal erotic language when it came to their desire for each other – would she be able to intuit what he was saying from his body language and tone of voice alone? Fundamentally, what she wanted to know was whether he wanted her enough to display obvious desire.

Another woman that I counseled with her husband had a fantasy that she wanted to rent horses and go out into a meadow, where she would take off all her clothes and ride naked like Lady Godiva as her husband watched her. This was an enormously busy working mother who felt her identity had been subsumed by her many duties. She wanted to feel carefree and to once again be an alive spirit in her husband's eyes.

Another couple that came to see me discussed the husband's fantasy. "I fantasize about taking advantage of you when you're asleep," he confessed to his wife. His fantasy was for her to feign unconsciousness. He wanted to experience domination, with her giving no resistance or aid. Men who have domination fantasies are usually men who feel subordinate in other areas of their lives; they feel stepped on and want to experience power.

Erotic fantasies are often a window not just into your spouse's erotic mind but into his or her psyche. They can lead to very valuable discussions that help you get to know each other better. The effect spills out into the rest of life. Fantasies reveal much about the subconscious – that's why they're so individual.

Should you indulge such fantasies? Should you share them with your spouse? What if you tell your spouse your fantasy and he or she rejects it and thinks it's infantile? While there is always a risk that these kinds of revelations may involve pain, isn't *not* telling your spouse about your inner erotic mind more dangerous? Doesn't it betray an absence of honesty and intimacy? Eroticism is by its very nature dangerous. Life is like that. People who aren't willing to take risks may shelter themselves from big losses, but they also miss out on big wins.

This brings me to an important point about eroticism: it's

not meant to be cozy and cuddly. Lust means lovemaking that is passionate, raw, vigorous, and almost violent in its intensity.

Not all lovemaking is meant to be tender and gentle. It's also not only about the intimate emotional connection. Sometimes it's just about raw desire and lust. That's part of the point of the Jewish system that separates a husband and wife for about twelve days out of every month: it's about the kind of lovemaking that ensues when you have been separated for twelve days. It's not tender; on the contrary it's deeply passionate.

Eroticism is by its very nature dangerous. Life is like that. People who aren't willing to take risks may shelter themselves from big losses, but they also miss out on big wins.

And it's clearly meant to be so. After twelve days apart, do you think the law mandates a slow, gradual reconnection in gentle, progressive steps? Not at all: the reunion night is a complete and abrupt return to full intimacy, with all the urgency of two weeks of accumulated hunger and passion.

If Judaism wanted sex that is only intimate, soft, and tender, then there's no way it would mandate sex on the night of a wedding. Jewish law mandates no physical contact between a couple before the wedding night. Wouldn't you think the law would be that now that you are permitted to each other, you should start by holding hands one night, the next night you should kiss, and so on, in a gradual establishment of intimate contact? But this is not how it works. Suddenly, on the wedding night, you're expected to have sex. Why? Because it's about lust. The couple has pent-up lust for each other and that lust ought to be expressed. You can't call that emotionally intimate. You can't call that loving. It's pure, unadulterated passion. It's about wanting someone so deeply that you can't hold back.

Erica Jong touched a chord in her iconic 1973 novel *Fear of Flying* when she coined the term "zipless" to describe a sexual encounter free of hindrances or complications, without commitment or emotional attachment. She was talking about an experience of pure lust, and many women really responded to it. Most women don't actually crave such an experience with a stranger, but why not have such an experience with your spouse? You can cuddle and be tender afterwards, but in the moment, why not give in to wild abandon and a pure experience of raw, primal lust?

It is my opinion that the greatest bulwark against infidelity is erotic satisfaction in marriage. This grants you an internal immunity. By bringing sinful pleasure into your marriage, you inoculate your relationship against actual transgression. Keep your lust for each other instead of being warm and fuzzy with each other and lusting after someone else.

Chapter 8

The Paradox of Trust

The Essential Contradiction

One of the many contradictions of life is the paradox of trust in marriage. The common wisdom is that trust in a marriage is essential. And there's an element of truth to that. How would love thrive in a relationship that had no trust? At the same time, however, trust is the enemy of passion. To trust completely that your spouse is yours and would never cheat on you is tantamount to believing that your spouse is not attractive to others and – even worse – is not a fully sexual person with his or her own erotic impulses and interests. It is within this paradox that the key to sustaining long-term lust in a marriage lies.

A *New York Times* article about the pervasive problem of waning female sexual desire highlighted a fascinating point:

One theory holds that it's a challenge for both sexes to maintain passion over the long-term because it's threatening to desire the same person from whom we seek security and true understanding. It leaves us feeling too vulnerable. As Stephen A. Mitchell, one of the leaders of relational psychoanalysis, described it: "Sustaining desire for something important from someone important is the central danger of emotional life. What is so dangerous about desiring someone you have is that you can lose him or her."[97]

We want two things out of the same person that cannot coexist. A marriage is based on love, trust, devotion, and dedication. We look to our spouses for stability in our lives. At the same time we want to be excited, passionate, and full of desire. In a trusting relationship, however, trust becomes the enemy of desire. You become complacent and bored. There's total predictability; your spouse is already won over – there's no thrill of the chase. Furthermore, if your spouse can be completely trusted, the implication is that he or she is not desirable to or desirous of others but only totally devoted to you. To have 100 percent trust in your spouse would mean you are convinced that your spouse is ordinary and has no other options – what could be more of a cold shower on a relationship?

Conversely, when you greatly desire someone, it's tremendously exciting but it also puts you in a painful position. Will the desire be reciprocated? You need the other person; your desire puts you in a weak position. The other person is in a position to be able to hurt you. When the person you desire is your spouse, the source of your security, it's frightening to put yourself in this position. So you start turning the desire off, to keep yourself from being hurt, to safeguard yourself from the vulnerability of desire. A husband may fear exploring his wife's erotic mind in the fullest, because seeing her as a fully sensual woman will open him up to doubt and pain that he cannot fully possess her – her very sexuality poses a challenge to his ego. The way husbands deal with that problem all too often is by silently and subconsciously extinguishing their wives' libidos. Women also may be the ones who cut off deep intimacy. One out of three women have been sexually abused in some way. That becomes a very big obstacle to intimacy, as women who have been abused don't trust men, don't allow them all the way in, even after marriage.

> Lust awakens an essential contradiction. We want security, stability, and trust on the one hand and eroticism, unpredictability, and overwhelming desire on the other.

Lust awakens an essential contradiction. You can't have complete trust for your spouse because total security in your relationship characterizes your spouse as fundamentally undesirable and asexual, extinguishing your desire. Yet a complete absence of trust is shattering, leaving you vulnerable to unimaginable pain.

Keith came to see me about his marriage. He and Michelle had been husband and wife for ten years, and had two kids. Although Keith was generally a good guy, and he loved Michelle, he had already succumbed to three affairs. One affair lasted two months. He had two more affairs spaced three years apart with two married women. He didn't really know why he'd done it – when he looked back he couldn't pinpoint the cause. He could certainly pinpoint the effect, however, which had been fast and furious since Michelle had found out what he'd done.

They say hell hath no fury like a woman scorned, and Michelle was looking to prove it. She hated him for what he'd done. She took a marker and blackened his face out of all the family photos, called all her friends and told them what he did. She was furious beyond words (although there had been plenty of those). And Keith didn't really understand the depth of her rage. "Fine," he said to me, "what I did was wrong, but look how cold and horrible she is."

"Think about it from her perspective," I told Keith. "Marriage for a woman is an awful deal when you look at it on the surface. She has to give up her name and identity. She has to have the babies and have her body permanently altered. Women, in this sexist and ageist society, are said to age more quickly than men, often have to hold down two jobs (employment outside the house plus chief responsibility for the domestic work and childcare), etc., etc. So why do they do it? Why do women get married? A woman wants to be special, to feel unique. She wants her uniqueness corroborated by a man who places her at the center of his existence, who makes her his one and only. Like the first two of the Ten Commandments: primacy and exclusivity. The one and the only.

"You're wondering why your wife is so angry and so mean to you. She made all the sacrifices that every woman makes to get married, and you deprived her of the one thing she was supposed to get. She was supposed to be the center of your existence and live without rivals. So she's bitter. And the worst thing is that you aren't even acknowledging the pain you caused her. It's one thing to cause the pain, but it's another thing not to even acknowledge it. That's why she hates you so much. You don't get it? Well, my friend, she's going to make you get it for the rest of your life. She's going to make your kids hate you, your friends hate you; she will do everything she can to wake you up to what you did to her, because you are asleep."

People get married to feel special. When your spouse is giving that special feeling to someone else instead, it's devastating. This can include looking at pornographic images of others, or thinking about someone else while making love. Jewish values actually recognize this kind of mental infidelity – thinking about someone other than your spouse during intimacy – as a grave transgression, and it is forbidden in Jewish law.

You have to maintain some level of distrust of your spouse's total fidelity to you, lest you relegate him or her to the category of nonsexual being. On the other hand when you really undermine trust in the relationship, you destroy the foundation. A serious breach in trust in a marriage can be tremendously difficult to repair; there's always that doubt. You don't want to be dependent on someone who has hurt you so deeply.

> *Alyssa is smart, balanced, and successful, with a prominent professional job. She really loved Brett, but when she discovered he'd had an affair on her, she left immediately. Brett had a hard time accepting the breakup. For months afterwards he would call and write her constantly, begging for her forgiveness. But Alyssa was immovable. "I'm a forgiving person," she said, "but I can never take him back." When I asked her what made her resolve so ironclad, she said, "Because when someone does that, it changes the very nature of the relationship; it can never be what it was. I can't forgive him because it will never be the same."*

I actually consider Alyssa's view somewhat extreme. With a lot of love and forbearance, some couples surmount an episode of infidelity and go on to rebuild their relationship. Yet Alyssa's point is well taken. Infidelity can never be completely undone. It can be forgiven but not forgotten.

In my experience of counseling couples, there's nothing as painful as the loss of trust. It destroys love and it destroys desire. The loss of trust that results from infidelity of all types is positively soul-destroying. The highest validation of your worth and desirability is when someone takes him or herself off the market to a couple of billion other marriageable men or women in the world and chooses *you*. What could be worse than being made to feel utterly ordinary by the person who's supposed to make you feel the most special (and once did)? When your boss fires you, that makes you feel very ordinary and it really hurts, but he only ever owned the things that you did; he never owned *who you were*. When your boss fires you, he's not rejecting your core personhood; he's rejecting your performance. He never owned you; he only owned your work product. So getting fired is not a rejection of your core self. When your spouse rejects you, it feels like a rejection of the essence of who you are. It confirms your own inner fear of inadequacy: *maybe I'm really not good enough, maybe in the final analysis I don't matter.*

> *Mary was married to Stuart for ten years when he had an affair with a woman he met on an airplane. When she found out, Mary would not be consoled. She insisted on leaving. I tried to calm her down, urging her to give her marriage a chance. "No," she said. "Knowing he lusted after someone else, even if he didn't love her, has changed the way I see Stuart. It's not the same. I don't feel he's mine and I don't feel he wants me. I can't live with him anymore." She refused to be mollified and she left.*

Love and trust are the water of a relationship. Lust and jealousy are the fire. Without love and trust, a marriage withers.

Without fire, it is cold. Both are needed, yet how can they coexist? We want security, stability, and trust on the one hand and eroticism, lust, and passion on the other. How can we get both those things from the same person when fire and water can't coexist?

> You are a garden fountain, a well of flowing water streaming down from Lebanon. (Song of Songs 4:15)
>
> Love...burns like blazing fire, like a mighty flame. (Song of Songs 8:6)

Jewish law gives us a glimpse at the beginnings of an answer when it mandates a monthly period of separation. Husband and wife live about half the month as lovers, and the other half as celibate, yet loving companions. Half the month is fire, half is water. But the truth is that the two categories don't split so neatly. The celibate part of the month feeds the passionate by allowing lust to grow during the time apart. The passionate part of the month feeds the comfort and security because of the closeness that follows intimacy. Fire and water do coexist.

Maimonides famously advised following the "golden mean." A lot of people think he was talking about compromise, finding a point somewhere in the middle. Compromise is a passionless idea. Compromises are generally forced on you out of necessity, and neither side is truly happy. Maimonides' beautiful idea of the golden mean is not compromise; rather, it's the synthesis of opposites that can never be fully reconciled. It's a totally different concept. There is no resolution to the dichotomy of the fire and water of marriage, the need for trust and love and coziness on one side, and jealousy and lust and discomfort on the other. Don't try to resolve that tension. Embrace it. Live with it.

Embracing the contradiction takes a lot of practice, but it can be done. Think of a great athlete. What's the hardest thing about reaching athletic greatness? It's the day of the competition. You worked for four years for the Olympics, and now it's the day of the race – the hundred-meter sprint. Four years of grueling practice, and the whole thing is going to be decided in ten seconds. And on top of that, there are two billion people watching. That's tension! The great athlete is the person who actually thrives on that tension, without trying to reconcile it. The great athlete drinks in the audience, tastes the four years of work, embraces the ten-second challenge, and fixes everything into one burst of creative tension.

Creative tension is not the same thing as anxiety. Anxiety is where you bottle up the tension and it has no outlet. Creativity is where the tension actually frees you. In a marriage, productive creative tension comes from radical honesty. Together, with great openness, you have to learn to strike the correct balance of trust. You have to distrust your spouse enough to acknowledge his or her essential sexuality and desirability to others and your need to continuously woo each other. And you have to trust your spouse enough to know that notwithstanding his or her attraction to others, the love and devotion in the marriage (not to mention your spouse's commitment to morality) will safeguard fidelity. Through that trust you learn to open a path to deep erotic exploration. This is a tension that you cannot reconcile. You have to embrace it.

The Positive Power of Jealousy

Jealousy gets a bad rap in our culture today, but the fact is that a little bit of jealousy is essential in marriage. To be completely without jealousy would indicate that you see your spouse as a person who has no attractiveness to others and no sensual nature that would imply a possibility of being attracted to others. A little distrust is an indication that there is eroticism inherent in the relationship.

We saw earlier how the patriarch Abraham and matriarch Sarah kept lust alive in their marriage with a healthy amount of distance between them, as evidenced by Abraham's comment as they descend to Egypt: "Behold, I now know that you're a beautiful woman" (Genesis 12:11). Abraham is convinced that Pharaoh is going to see Sarah and take her away. But is Abraham also afraid that Sarah actually might gravitate toward a powerful man who wants her? "Say you are my sister," he enjoins her, "so that I will be treated well for your sake and my life will be spared because of you" (Genesis 12:13). The original text reveals something interesting about Abraham's request: "*Imri na, achoti at*" (Say, I beg of you, that you are my sister). He's pleading with her: perhaps he doesn't fully trust her in that moment? Pharaoh is a powerful man, after all – what if she will really be tempted? It's certainly very flattering to a woman that the most powerful man in the world wants you.

I have a friend whose wife had an affair with a world-renowned businessman. It was beyond soul-destroying. He felt utterly emasculated, like there was no way he could compete. I spent much time trying to restore his sense of self. It's bad enough when a spouse is unfaithful. It's much worse when the person your spouse has an affair with is someone whom you feel – rightly or wrongly – is out of your league.

Faced with the threat of a mighty ruler's interest in his wife, Abraham takes nothing for granted. He does not assume that he fully possesses Sarah. He sees her as a beautiful woman and knows that Pharaoh will, too. And furthermore he realizes that Sarah has passions of her own that could be inflamed when she is placed in a situation of being admired by a powerful man. Abraham models a healthy level of jealousy in a passionate marriage. Noticing the attractiveness of your spouse to others at all times is painful, and involves a certain level of distrust, but it also allows for the flourishing of passion in the marriage.

The Bible contains another fascinating episode that reveals the power of correctly balanced and directed distrust in a marriage. In Numbers 5:11–31, we are instructed regarding the *sotah*, a wife suspected of being unfaithful. If a woman has been seen to have secluded herself with another man, and the husband warned her not to do this again but she did,[98] and "feelings of jealousy come over her husband and he suspects his wife" (Numbers 5:14), then a mystifying public ritual is to be performed. The man brings his wife to the priest in the Temple, and the priest mixes earth from the Temple floor into sacred water. After uncovering the woman's hair (an indication of her immodesty in secluding herself with another man, since married women are required to cover their hair), the priest informs her that drinking these bitter waters will reveal her guilt or innocence. If she drinks the waters and she is innocent, no harm will befall her. If she is guilty of adultery, however, she will suffer immediate death.

If the woman agrees to the test (she may also refuse, in which case she and her husband must be divorced[99]), the priest then writes relevant Bible verses on a parchment,

> Noticing the attractiveness of your spouse to others at all times is painful, and involves a certain level of distrust, but it also allows for the flourishing of passion in the marriage.

dissolves the ink into the water, and gives it to her to drink. If she is guilty, she will then die a gruesome death.[100] If she is innocent, however, not only will she not be harmed, but the couple will be reconciled and she will be blessed with fertility (even if she was infertile before), giving birth easily to beautiful children (even if her previous children were unattractive). Finally, after her innocence is proven, her husband is instructed that he has full permission to resume intimate relations with her.[101]

This episode is strongly emphasized, described at a level of detail that is somewhat unusual in the Bible text. (By way of comparison, the test of the unfaithful wife extends across twenty lengthy verses, while the Ten Commandments are enumerated in Exodus 20:1–14 and Deuteronomy 5:6–18[102] in thirteen or fourteen very brief ones.) Let's take note of the fact that there is no biblical passage about the devoted wife, the faithful wife – no ceremony where she is honored, or the like. On the contrary there is this lengthy passage on the possibly unfaithful wife, making her the most famous archetypal wife in the Hebrew Bible.

The test of the wayward wife of course has derogatory aspects: she's going to be humiliated in front of her community; she may die (if she is guilty). But it also ends in a potential blessing: if she is proven innocent, trust will be restored to her marriage, and she will be blessed with particularly special children. This woman who brings out a certain passion in her husband is in a certain sense a blessing. The very fact that her husband is jealous and worried about her behavior with other men shows that he has passion for her. Her sensuality is emphasized in the uncovering of her hair, which is considered a deeply erotic feminine attribute.

Another fascinating aspect of this episode is the erasure
of God's name in the course of the ritual. Jewish law forbids
the erasure of God's name, yet it is specifically commanded
by God in the test of the possibly unfaithful wife. Why does
God not only permit but command the erasure of His own
name in this ritual? Because the purpose of the ritual is to
allay the husband's doubts and restore the intimate relationship between husband and wife, and this is a cause for which
God willingly lends His name. As the nineteenth-century
sage Samson Raphael Hirsch wrote in his commentary on
Numbers, the episode of the wayward wife "shows the Presence of God in every Jewish married life, the faithfulness to
each other of husband and wife as the quite special object of
God's attention...."

This whole episode reinforces the priority placed on the
intimate marital relationship and on properly directed lust
within marriage. The wayward wife has defied her husband
and given him serious cause for jealousy by putting herself
in a compromised position with a man. Yet she is not punished for this. If she has in fact committed adultery, refuses
to confess, and agrees to submit to the test, she will indeed
receive the ultimate punishment (and commentaries also
indicate that the man with whom she committed adultery
will himself suffer the same fate if she dies in the test of the
bitter waters). But if her seclusion with another man was only
an indiscretion and she did not actually commit adultery, she
does not merely walk away unpunished, but she actually is
rewarded with blessing.

While it's true that the wayward wife has behaved in-
discreetly and has thereby caused marital turmoil and pain,
her essential nature as a passionate, vibrant, irrepressible,

seductive woman is not only not punished but is actually blessed. In this passage, God explicitly endorses the passionate woman in the expression of her core femininity. Her passionate nature is not to be suppressed, but merely properly directed. Her husband is enjoined to resume his intimate relationship with her; he should be her partner in passionate intensity, not leaving her alone searching for one. God endorses passion and lust, when it is properly directed within marriage.

The episode of the wayward wife shows us how jealousy in a marriage can in fact be a sign of blessing: it is precisely because this couple has a fiery, passionate relationship that the issue came up. But it also acknowledges that when trust is excessively compromised, healthy marital intimacy cannot continue until trust is restored. Indeed, once the wife has been labeled as a suspected adulteress, the marital relationship is actually forbidden until her innocence is proven.[103]

> Craig was convinced that he was not the father of his youngest child, as he suspected his wife Allison of having been unfaithful with one of his closest friends. Allison swore she was innocent and wanted to arrange for a paternity test but Craig wouldn't let her because he was too afraid of the results. They remained married but totally celibate because there was no trust. Craig couldn't be with her because he couldn't bring himself to believe in her.

There has to be a balance. When there is no trust, there can be no real intimacy. But jealousy – a lack of complete trust – is essential to a vibrant lustful relationship because only in this context do you see your spouse as a desirable and desirous sensual person whose sexual and erotic needs must constantly be addressed. Jealousy is based on insecurity: you're only jealous over your spouse if there's a possibility of losing him or her. The very possibility of that loss reinforces your desire to hold onto your spouse. Jealousy is about staking your claim, asserting your territory.

> *Allen and Joan came for counseling. Throughout our initial session, every time Allen wanted to make a point he would touch Joan's elbow or pat her shoulder. Joan's body language showed that Allen's touch was really irritating her. I immediately knew what the trouble was in this marriage. Joan had stopped loving her husband with the same intensity as before. Allen clearly suspected as much and he was very insecure about it. He wanted to show possession by touching Joan, as if to say, I can touch her in public whenever I want. She belongs to me. She's mine. But Joan didn't want to be touched. If she had really loved him she'd have been flattered that he was tactile. That was the telltale sign that told me everything I needed to know: Allen wanted to be possessive, but Joan didn't want to be possessed because she did not reciprocate the same level of affection.*

In a relationship that has depth and passion, a proper amount of jealousy and possessiveness demonstrates erotic attraction and is welcomed by the spouse who feels validated by the attention and by the recognition of his or her intrinsic attractiveness and sensual nature.

Going Deeper with Trust

People love variety. Men especially love sexual variety. Men who aren't experiencing variety in their intimate relationships become bored, and this is a major challenge in long-term relationships. There are actually two kinds of variety, however, and most people only tap into one of them. There's vertical variety and there's horizontal variety. Horizontal variety is basically surface deep. Sexually it manifests as different partners, or different acts with the same partner. It can often be very superficial. When you're tired of one woman you switch to another. When you're tired of one position you try another. This can be fun, and every relationship needs a little bit of it, like trying a new spice in the kitchen, but there's no depth here.

Vertical exploration, on the other hand, means going on the one hand deeper and on the other hand higher with the same person, plumbing the depths and soaring with the highs. And for this kind of erotic exploration you have to have a solid basis of trust. No one wants to reveal his or her deepest self to someone who can't be trusted.

Serious depth can be intimidating. In general, most people have a tendency to want to shy away from intensity. We've talked about how Americans tend to want to extinguish rather than explore tension and seek a pacifying comfort, even at the cost of deadening themselves with mind-numbing agents like drugs, alcohol, or television. Vertical exploration is definitely not comfortable. We tend to fear emotional nakedness and vulnerability. We'd rather stay on the level of horizontal erotic exploration because it's so much more comfortable – it doesn't penetrate to our core.

Horizontal variety is often found in sex toys and a million and one different contortionist positions... all of which demand nothing from you emotionally and distract you from a real, face-to-face encounter. The missionary position is often scorned as a plain "vanilla" experience. In actuality, many people may be intimidated by the intimate potential of this position because it is a full-out commitment: full-body contact, face to face, the closest you can get. In truth, missionary is possibly the best venue for vertical exploration, but most people will try to defuse the intensity of it by closing their eyes and avoiding gazing into each other's souls. The vast majority of women can't reach climax with their eyes open. They say the reason is that no wife wants to see her husband having such a good time. But to get serious, the intensity of peering into the infinite of each other's personalities during sex is intimidating for most people. Most people therefore close their eyes during orgasm, retreating into a world of private fantasy and stimuli but thereby shutting off the even more powerful stimulus of witnessing their partner achieve total psychological and spiritual nakedness.

Horizontal exploration shouldn't be discounted either. When you do make the effort to explore your spouse vertically, you'll find that it leads back to the horizontal as well, as even your spouse's fingers become of interest to you. When Moses sent spies to get to know the Land of Israel (Numbers 13:17–20), he directed them to explore every last inch of it: you have to love the whole land, in all its aspects.

Think of an explosive erotic connection as a pressure cooker. In order to build up an effective pressure, you have to keep the lid closed – you can't let steam escape. If you're always opening the lid, you'll never reach the explosive rocking pressure. Allowing your erotic attention to escape outside your marriage through horizontal exploration of other people (including porn and even masturbation) prevents you from having the explosive erotic connection that really gets things cooking. Put another way, if you're always snacking, always finding ways to appease your hunger, you're not going to be hungry for the full meal that would really satisfy you.

An electrifying erotic relationship with your spouse carries with it an intensity and a holiness that may sometimes make you uncomfortable. It demands something from you. You have to show up for it, with an emotional presence and a level of commitment that do not come easily. But this is the key to keeping lust alive in the long term: making a total commitment to the primacy and exclusivity of your spouse keeps all the steam in the relationship. Commitment is the ultimate key to sustaining erotic fulfillment, because making a complete and total commitment to your spouse creates the environment in which total erotic exploration can occur.

In an atmosphere of trust, husbands and wives can start to have the erotic conversations that are the basic building blocks of an erotic relationship. First of all, having erotic conversations with your spouse, in and of itself, stimulates desire. The more you speak about desire, the more you desire. It's the flip side of the concept expressed in a common rule of anger management that if you want to control your temper you need to not talk about things that anger you. Speaking about feelings fans the flames of those feelings. So once you're talking together about your erotic relationship, you're already starting down the right path.

> Commitment is the ultimate key to sustaining erotic fulfillment, because making a complete and total commitment to your spouse creates the environment in which total erotic exploration can occur.

Most people, if they engage in erotic conversation at all, however, stop at horizontal exploration: I like when you touch me here, or kiss me in this way. Speaking with your spouse about what attracts you, what really pleasures you, is a central element of every good marriage. But there's more: you can go really deep into vertical exploration and strip away the externalities to speak about the motivations, the causes. That is, not just what your spouse's fantasy or fetish is, but *why*. When you analyze together what lies beneath your erotic inclinations, you can tap into a tremendous wellspring of connection, touching not just on your erotic interests but on who you are as people and on what motivates you.

> *Christina is a pious woman from an evangelical Christian family. She works for an international company that arranges conferences overseas, and her job involves a lot of travel. Lately she's going through a stage that's confusing to her and her husband, Dan. She doesn't know why she's doing this, but she's been dressing more provocatively and acting more flirtatiously with other men. She seems to crave male attention and she puts a lot more time into her appearance than she used to. Once upon a time Christina would use extra mileage to bring Dan along with her on her business trips, but she doesn't do that anymore. She's much more adventurous than he is and when she travels abroad for business, it really bothers him. He thinks that she quietly resents him because they never had kids.*
>
> *In the course of speaking with Christina, we uncovered the fact that something inside of her is pushing her as she gets older toward a need for more and more attention. I discovered that this traces back to her youth. She was raised to be more than anything else a good girl, in an evangelical Christian family in a mega-church. Christina's relationship with her father was basically "yes, sir." Christina married a nice, sweet guy, and she lived all her life as a quiet, shy, good girl, until one day she woke up and said, "This is not satisfying."*

Christina wanted more. Most of all she wanted more attention, and especially from the opposite sex. She's very good at her job and she gets a lot of validation from it. More and more of the business leaders for whom she arranges trips depend on her, rely on her, bring her along with them on these trips. But also, they like her. It's all innocent, but they like her. She's thriving on the attention and she never knew why. She was really deprived of it as a child. She was really never given unconditional validation. She was supposed to be a good girl and always volunteer for other people. She always had to do things to get her father's approval, and now when she sits and laughs and lets go, and she sees that men enjoy her company, she finds she can just BE for the first time in her life.

Dan, Christina's husband, feels a bit left out. He doesn't understand this core need for attention. He doesn't get it. Now, can Dan give it to her? Will she always need other men? The truth is that we always need a little bit of attention from other people. It's where that dependency on others begins to encroach on our essential connection to our spouses that our marriages are eroded. Time will tell whether Dan can step up to the plate to change their relationship and create a more intense connection, but understanding what makes Christina tick is a meaningful step in the right direction.

People are constantly evolving, growing, changing. Women especially feel stifled in relationships when men don't want them to grow, or actually impede their growth. Women in general are much more in tune with the vastness of the universe. In Kabbalah a woman is a circle, while a man is a line. When two men get together they tend to talk about linear subjects such as sports, politics, money, women (in a linear fashion, i.e., 36-24-36), and electronics. Women on the other hand talk about relationships and shopping: a circle of intimacy and a circle of acquisition (the latter comes to substitute for the former when the former is impoverished). As Audrey Nelson and Claire Damken Brown report in their *Gender Communication Handbook*: "The topics of conversation chosen by men tend to be 'safe' topics, such as work, sports and financial matters. Men's speech tends to revolve around external things and usually involves factual communication, not feelings or inner thoughts. In contrast, women will incorporate more person-centered topics and initiate interpersonal matters. Their speech is more apt to deal with feelings than men's topics of conversation."[104]

Men have to learn to follow women's example to enter into a circle of intimacy with their wives. This requires some emotional work because men in our culture are trained to be strong. Men don't even tell their wives when they get laid off from a job, let alone that they feel emotionally dependent on their wives. Men don't want to show that they're vulnerable. Furthermore, all the studies show that women look up to men who are confident: that's the sexiest quality of a man for women.[105] So on the one hand, women want men to confess their emotional dependency and connectedness and utter dependence ("I need you"), and on the other hand that shows weakness. Men are supposed to go out and fight and be a woman's warrior, and if a man confesses his vulnerability to his wife, she may be wondering, how could someone who needs me so badly protect me as well? So a woman has to live with that contradiction. And a man has to get beyond the macho demeanor and stop worrying, *does my wife see me as someone who's strong?* Ultimately there's no complete resolution to these contradictions: we have to embrace them and even thrive on the tension they create. And isn't that what marriage is, after all – embracing the contradiction between the masculine and the feminine?

American life hates contradictions. We don't want to embrace contradictions, so we've created a unisex society in which men and women are as similar as possible. But this destroys eroticism and passion. In the same way we've created an unhealthy American society based on fast food, instant gratification that knocks out hunger. Hunger is about embracing the contradiction: If I'm hungry, why don't I eat? Well, there are good reasons not to satisfy your hunger. You're supposed to live with that contradiction. You're meant to embrace hunger. That's the essence of this book. To live erotically with kosher lust is to embrace the contradiction of the masculine and the feminine, of trust versus jealousy, of needing someone on whom you base your stability.

Learning to live with that kind of tension, internalizing it, and turning it into a creative force – that's the key to a life of long-lasting passion.

Chapter 9

Flesh of My Flesh: A Return to Eden

The Goal-Oriented Approach

A woman wrote to me from New Mexico asking for counseling for her and her husband by phone. She was 29 and her husband 31. Married for three years, she said she was unhappy and they were drifting apart. On the phone together, I asked them about their intimate life. He bragged, "We have sex three times a week. I'm really attracted to my wife." She interjected, "Yeah, and it lasts three minutes. It's very goal oriented." This is something I hear from wives constantly. Even if the frequency of sex in the marriage is high, its duration is quite short. We can blame men but ultimately we have to blame orgasm.

What has most killed off sex in America is, paradoxically, that aspect of sex which is supposed to make it so pleasurable, namely the orgasm. Sex in America is almost entirely goal oriented. It's not about the journey but the destination, not an act of exploration but a rush to the finish line.

This is a cultural phenomenon perhaps best illustrated by a commercial for a popular personal lubricant in which the busy and distracted couple tells the audience that the product helps them "get to the good stuff" faster.

With the search for the all-powerful orgasm dominating American sexuality, sexual climax has actually become an impediment to intimacy and lust.

For men, having an orgasm means losing most of their interest in sex. The orgasm purges their bodies of erotic desire. The effect can be quite startling. One moment he is in the throes of passion, telling his wife how much he wants her, his hunger for her insatiable. The very next moment he is lifeless, having lost the desire to even converse. He is numb. He is unconscious. One moment he is shouting from the rooftops how much he desires her, and the next moment she's wondering whether she should call the undertaker.

The finish line has been reached, the goal achieved. It is only sleep he craves. The French recognize this phenomenon in their euphemism for orgasm; they call it *la petite mort*, "the little death."

For women orgasm is problematic for precisely the opposite reason: in marital sex they have so few of them. Studies show that only one-quarter of women report that they "always" climax during intercourse.[106] As time goes on, a woman begins to enjoy sex less and less, not only because pleasurable sexual release is denied her but because sex is over so quickly that she ends up feeling used rather than pleasured.

Ironically, in this context sex divides rather than unites the couple. His climax puts an instant end to his desire. This kind of mechanical interaction may involve pleasure – however fleeting – but it is experienced solo; it separates each participant back into his or her own world, rather than uniting them in a shared transcendent experience.

One of the reasons we are having such unsatisfying orgasms these days is that we're not sufficiently focused on one another. Our lust for our spouses is being lost. Our sexuality is diffused and dissipated, focused too much on multiple targets to achieve the laser-like focus required to achieve oneness.

Indeed, if we don't focus intently during sex, we can't climax at all. More than anything else, orgasm requires not stimulation but mental concentration. Indeed, in its highest, finest form orgasm is a moment of pure presence. It crystallizes all of our being into the here-and-now, giving us the pleasure of what we in our multi-tasking world today so lack: intensity.

> In its highest, finest form orgasm is a moment of pure presence.

Please note: if you are having problems with persistent impotence, pain during sex, loss of libido not remedied by increased focus on the relationship, a history of sexual abuse, or other such medical or emotional issues, please seek assistance from a qualified professional. Medical treatment or counseling may be indicated.

Orgasm has the potential to be the ultimate intensity, but it doesn't always work out that way, because there isn't just one type of orgasm. In fact, there are three, corresponding to the three types of lust: material, emotional, and spiritual.

1. The material orgasm. This is a biological-hormonal climax, centered in the body. It is purely a matter of muscular contractions. The sexual partner is almost an afterthought: it could be anyone. Or no one. People can achieve this kind of climax through sexual toys or masturbating to pornography. An orgasm like this is a depersonalized connection that may allow physical pleasure and relaxation but does not foster any sort of intimacy.

2. The emotional orgasm. This is a mental-psychological climax, centered in the mind. This is a far more intimate erotic experience in which you are mentally focused on the person you're with. Orgasm propels you, together, to a higher state of awareness. People describe an expansion of consciousness and heightened sensations. As you soar higher with the person you love, you experience a lightness of being occasioned by a burst of color and sound. As your mental horizon expands, you experience reality with a feeling of sheer presence. You are amazed at how powerful the sensations of the world can be. Colors become brighter. Light is more intense. Sounds became symphonic. There is an elevation of the physical: the natural becomes miraculous and the everyday unique. The bonding force of this type of orgasm is incredible, its adhesive quality lingering well after orgasm has ceased. You drink each other in through every cell of the body. As you lose yourself through the stimulus of another person, you are slowly grafted onto each other's souls.

3. The spiritual orgasm. This is a metaphysical-spiritual climax, centered in the soul. The body sloughs away completely and the sexual detonation transforms the body into pure spirit. You no longer feel hands and feet. You are energy itself. You become one with all that is around you, especially the person you love with whom you've shared the experience. You have visions of an infinite expanse of which you are a part, a blissful Eden-like world where everything is one and nothing is separate or divided. The mystical orgasm has you joining a spirit world, a place not of bodies but of light. All that we are is fused together into the starburst of one ecstatic moment. The steady gaze of a husband into the eyes of his wife amid the passionate sexual encounter leads both of them to experience a form of hypnotic engagement. The spiritual climax leads to emotional openness, spiritual transcendence, and even, for some, mystical visions.

One way for men to achieve mystical-spiritual climax is by absorbing the Tantric secret of delaying orgasm, first by a few minutes and then by a few days, thereby increasing the erotic hunger that culminates later in cliffhanger orgasms in which one's spouse becomes the source of unimaginable pleasure. (See my books *Kosher Adultery* and *The Kosher Sutra* for more on this, including specific "kosher Tantric" exercises.) Porn, adultery, and all forms of non-intimate or nonexclusive interaction, by contrast, become unappealing and disappointing substitutes.

In an intense sexual encounter, husbands can discover their wives' deepest fantasies and mysteries, as all a woman's defenses thaw in the heat of sexual peak. Wives are, by nature, reticent about discussing sexual fantasies openly, even with their husbands, which rightly conforms with a woman's more modest nature. As the Bible says, "All the glory of the king's daughter lies within" (Psalms 45:13/14).[107] But during sexual climax the natural filter disappears and the window to a wife's erotic mind opens completely. The secrets that flow and the passionate articulation of deep erotic need in the moment of orgasm provide the sexual excitement that is so necessary for sustaining passion in marital sex.

At its core, orgasm is involuntary: the body is stimulated to the point of automatic response that cannot be suppressed. The body becomes one with the beat of life in a cosmic state of flow, culminating in a rhythmic explosion. It is an act of surrender where the pleasurable release of stored sexual pleasure can no longer be controlled or contained. Something larger than us begins to take over. In its wake we are powerless. The experience captures the human encounter with the infinite; we surrender to the *mysterium tremendum*, the grand unknown before which all is rendered inconsequential.

In that sense, part of its near-infinite power is how incredibly liberating it is. Orgasm is a moment of unsurpassed spiritual and emotional elasticity. The strict rigidity of the body loosens. We become supremely present in the moment. Indeed, orgasm is presence incarnate. We shut off all the outside noise that normally distracts us. We are here. Now. Focused and alive. In a state of flow. It may last for only a few seconds but in the face of such freedom and pleasure, time is suspended. During the moments of intense orgasm, time loses its linear quality. All existence is rolled into one. Surrounding us is total peace. All cares of the world, all thoughts, all ideas, all niggling irritants, are pushed out.

Today we all multi-task. We rarely focus on one thing. But the searing focus on a single idea through the intensity of orgasm is immensely pleasurable and can connect us like no other experience. We become a wave of energy. And as the boundaries and human limitations are pushed back, there exists the possibility of becoming so much more than we otherwise are.

This is what lends orgasm such a spiritual quality. It's the human experience of pushing back the boundaries that limit us. Some orgasms are so powerful that they have a surreal quality. Time and space vanish. Some forget where and who they are and many women report blacking out. An intoxicating quality overtakes us, yet we have imbibed no foreign substance. In an Einsteinian moment, the body's matter is being converted into pure energy.

There are, however, inward and outward orgasms. The former pulls you into yourself. The latter draws you out. The inward orgasm's focus is only on the experience of physical pleasure. The stimulation of sex leads to feelings of bliss and delight. Those feelings are made stronger by tuning the other person out, though he or she is responsible for the stimulation in the first place. There are two people in bed but they have separate, individualistic experiences. The inward orgasm involves intense focus of erotic thoughts, but not necessarily about your spouse. It is a separate experience from your partner's. Sex may be shared, but the orgasm is solitary. When it is over you are forced to ask your spouse, "How was it for you?" A bizarre question when you think about it, given that you have just engaged in the most intimate experience available to two human beings.

Then there is the outward orgasm, one that pulls you out of yourself and grafts you onto another human being. This type of orgasm is mutually engaging. There is a powerful, conscious erotic connection. You have intensely amorous thoughts about the person you're with. You peer deeply into each other's eyes. At the moment of climax you feel your spirit leaving your body and entering another person. You experience a merging of souls to create a single erotic personality. This is the mystical concept of spiritual penetration, which is much more profound and unifying than physical penetration. In the moment of spiritual penetration a husband's interest is not in mere physical penetration but in invading her entire personality and becoming one. And what orgasm affords is a final loosening of the spirit, an unchaining of the self, which allows him to inhabit his wife in spirit, mind, and body, and she him.

Most people experience only the more limited, material, inward orgasm. You have sex with someone and in order to increase the mechanical stimulation you begin to tune the other person out. You close your eyes to focus on physical feelings. In your mind you begin to fantasize, perhaps even about someone else, an action that undermines the intimacy of the experience. You shut out all external noise and focus intently on the stimuli of sex. As you sink more deeply into yourself, your partner can no longer even read you. You now have two people whose bodies are having sex with each other but whose personalities are excluded from the experience. Their bodies are not in sync; there is an asymmetric rhythm that usually results in only one partner climaxing. The purpose of sex is intimacy, but this act has little.

Outward orgasm, however challenging, is what we must aim for. It involves powerful mental erotic stimulation that makes you so much more intimate with your spouse. You feel your spirit exiting yourself and entering into the other. Spiritual penetration trumps physical penetration. Most important for a woman is the feeling that a man desires her so deeply that he stimulates her to the point of ecstasy. He wants to see her transformed through his intense focus on her pleasure. He makes eye contact as he arouses her, creating a powerful erotic connection.

Outward orgasm loosens the fetters that imprison you; the differences between you dissolve. You are fully open to the healing power of intimacy and fully alive to passion's power. In this heightened state of intimacy you experience nonverbal communication. You begin to share feelings and emotions through the eyes alone. You feel a powerful electrical pulse passing between you, a spiritual current that is bringing you closer. You feel yourselves being joined as one. Time and space are suspended, which answers perhaps the most important question about sexual climax.

What? It's so short? A couple of seconds, and that's it?

That's the million-dollar question. Our society is sex-obsessed. Sex saturates our culture. And it turns out that the whole thing culminates in an experience that lasts but a few seconds. A few moments of pleasure is about all we can experience in life's most intense activity? Is that really as good as it gets? But the whole point of orgasm is that it transports you back to the eternity of Eden where there is no time or space. While there you rise above the space-time continuum. And though the physical experience may end abruptly in the body, its residue lingers in the soul. Even after you come down from the mountain's summit you are still able to internalize the experience. You know that Eden is a place that exists and you can begin to extrapolate beyond the confines of that momentary experience and make its effects last forever.

Every orgasmic finale to a loving sexual encounter between husband and wife is a return to Eden. You are no longer John and Sylvia. You are Adam and Eve.

Once, long ago in the mists of time, there were a man and a woman who were naked and bereft of everything but one another. They had no clothing, no house, no job, no car. But in each other they found paradise. Their desire was for each other and they felt no need to search for more. In the innocence of the sexual encounter they experienced a level of pleasure and bliss that we call Eden. The loving sexual encounter between husband and wife is what allows us to inhabit their identities, however momentarily. We lack for nothing; our only need is to hold the other. It doesn't have to be for much longer than a moment, because once we are there we know it exists and we spend our lives yearning and working to get back there. We lust for each other carnally in order to return to that sacred place. What matters is knowing that

> Every orgasmic finale to a loving sexual encounter between husband and wife is a return to Eden. You are no longer John and Sylvia. You are Adam and Eve.

at any moment, when the cares of the world overtake us, we can, together, lift off to paradise, bringing profound pleasure and happiness into our lives.

It's not the orgasm that is the goal but the state of transcendence that is achieved in the moment. Orgasm is not the end but the *means* to achieve something far greater.

Physical and Spiritual Transcendence

The Bible is so insightful in having no word for sex other than the word *knowledge*.

It's a mark of our time that sex has been so trivialized, coarsened, and vulgarized – made so utterly pedestrian – that married couples no longer feel its pull and are far more interested in watching television in the bedroom than rediscovering the soaring heights that only sex can bring.

To engage in the most passionate experience of sexual intimacy is to discover a level of yearning and transcendence in ourselves that we scarcely knew possible.

The passionate part is very important. It bridges the two sides of us that are often at war. By that I mean our souls and bodies. The body gravitates toward things of the earth and the soul toward more heavenly pursuits, the body toward materialism and the soul toward spirituality. The two are like wrestlers tied into a giant sack, forced to coexist but always as opponents, pushing outward in totally different directions.

Orgasm alone, out of all human experience, has the power to draw a man and a woman into each other's souls as they are drawn into each other's bodies, merging the physical and the spiritual. This is the power of the intimate marital bond.

The reason that sexual longing is so strong is that, at its core, it is the soul's desire to attach to another spirit. And that's why, amid its carnality, sex is so deeply spiritual. I am not the first author to point out the resonance of men and women so often screaming the name of God during orgasm; the spiritual component of the experience is inherent and innate. It's also the reason that the most magnetic and electrifying sex is when a husband and wife gaze into each other's eyes while they make love. The eyes are the windows to the soul and the soul begins to open completely. The interlocking of eyes is very difficult to sustain. But if you can fix your gaze without breaking the bond, you are teasing the soul out from its chamber. You are opening the window to each other's souls and becoming one spirit. Sexual congress brings together body and spirit so the two are no longer in conflict.

The highest point of sexual climax is where the spirit, mind, body, and soul are all synthesized. When a husband and wife connect in this way, they recapture an Eden-like state of ecstasy.

Adam and Eve existed in a paradise of spiritual and physical love. They were naked, they had no possessions, and yet they were content. Blissfully happy, in fact – satisfied in a way that is hard for us now to even imagine. Why? Because they had each other. All the splendors of the garden paled in comparison to the delight of being harmonized as one.

Their banishment from the garden came when they were no longer enough for each other, when they developed wants that were insatiable. The Serpent came to Eve and said, in essence: *What are you smiling for? How can you be content? How can you be satisfied when you don't even know what you're missing?* That's the meaning of pointing out the forbidden fruit to her. *Can you be happy when there are things you have not yet tasted or enjoyed? How do you know that the one thing that is forbidden to you wouldn't bring you levels of joy and pleasure you can scarcely dream of?*

Eve replied: *I have everything I need. There is nothing external that I need to complete me.* But the serpent sowed the seed of doubt: *How do you know there isn't something more? Maybe the pleasure of that one forbidden fruit is so great that it will eclipse everything you have known before....* So Eve began to focus not on what she had but rather on what she lacked. She began to yearn for an imagined happiness that seemed just out of reach, beckoning her from afar. Satisfaction was replaced with insatiability, contentment with unquenchable hunger, desire for her husband with desire for things. And it was the sowing of this unkosher lust that has led to such illicit longing and unhappiness throughout history. That is what destroys contentment: the suspicion that there is something better to be had, accompanied by an un-fillable chasm of desire. How many marriages have had the joy ripped right out of them because a husband stupidly yearns after another woman, or a wife after another man? Now you see why the Ten Commandments enjoins lusting after your own spouse and never someone else's. Lust and desire are absolutely vital in a marriage, but only when reserved for the person who is your soul mate and with whom you can share a deep spiritual and emotional – rather than just carnal – connection.

The sin of Adam and Eve was to imbibe the poison of the serpent, thereby becoming cold to all their blessings, including the blessing of having each other. Being together was no longer enough. They now wanted material objects, physical things, to make them happy.

But we can experience a temporary reversal of the expulsion from Eden; through our most intimate relationship we can recapture the primal state of bliss that is Eden, the supreme experience of intimacy that cancels out the noise of everything else, that experience of togetherness so intense that nothing else really matters.

The moment of climax, when reached through emotional togetherness and mutual engagement, has the power to transport you to this place of sheer presence. Nothing else exists for a couple in that moment. You are raised to a more elevated plane of human experience. You achieve a bond that pushes you into a single universe inhabited only by the two of you. External existence melts away and you are afforded a view of what life was like for Adam and Eve when they were alone with no other earthly inhabitants. They occupied a space in the world with no intrusions, no diversions, no distractions. Everything you could possibly want is already there. You can shut out the external world and be liberated from desire. With total focus on the current moment comes utter freedom.

Real delight in life comes from feeling emancipated. There is no pleasure like the feeling of liberation. And when you release all the pent-up sexual energy from your body, when you liberate the deep emotions of the heart, when lust and longing are given a safe arena to roam free and are completely focused on a loving and devoted target, the soul is set loose. You experience a level of physical and spiritual pleasure that lifts you to a different place. And seeing the world from that place, all the trivial, needling irritants fall by the wayside. You stop sweating the small stuff. Life feels grand; the body is at peace.

Orgasm puts all our material possessions, all our career ambitions, in perspective. We are not meant to take pleasure from objects, money, or status but from people in general and our beloved in particular. It is profound union with our spouse rather than winning the lottery that is supposed to make us feel like we're winners. We return to an Eden-like state by getting naked – shedding all the material possessions we think make us happy – and deriving pleasure from the liberated simplicity of the other's unadorned body.

The irony of this liberation is that the more bound you are to your partner, the more you experience freedom through your connection. It's specifically when you feel totally possessed, when you know that you're totally given over to someone, that you are able to liberate the pleasure and passion of the body, allowing the spirit to soar.

The Jewish sages commented poignantly on this contradiction of freedom through constriction nearly two millennia ago in *Pirkei Avot*, Ethics of the Fathers. Exodus 32:16 says, "*v'hamichtav michtav Elokim hu, charut al haluchot*" (the writing was the writing of God, engraved on the tablets). Ethics of the Fathers 6:2 comments, "Do not read *charut*, engraved, but rather *cherut*, freedom, for the only free person is one who studies Torah." The life of a religious Jew, bound by the commandments, is a life of liberation, of cleaving to God and His commandments. Likewise married life, bound to a spouse, consecrated to one person only, is a life in which one can experience the ultimate freedom. It is precisely the limitation and the exclusive focus of our sexuality and erotic desire on a single person that makes pleasure so intense and freedom so possible.

"This is now bone of my bones and flesh of my flesh," said Adam when he first saw Eve (Genesis 2:23). Those beautiful words of the Bible are realized in that supreme moment when we can slough away physical concerns and break through our individual spheres of isolation in order to truly connect with the one other person who loves us most in the world, the one person with whom we have total freedom of erotic expression.

Sexuality – and particularly intense orgasm – is an opportunity for self-discovery and knowledge of one's spouse like few other life experiences. During sexual climax the body, mind, and spirit are stripped completely bare. Inhibition melts away along with all basic mental furniture. Cognition is transmuted into sheer, raw emotion. A closed personality becomes utterly porous. The rigid pathways of the mind expand, the slits of the spirit open. We are able to see and absorb that to which we are normally blind. We experience an elasticity and expansion of the self that has the potential to leave us unlocked even after sex is over, if only we learn to cultivate its power.

In allowing her husband to be one with her, a wife is capable of transporting him back through time and space to a place that removes all pain and sorrow. A place that is hidden and removed. Covered and inaccessible. It's a place that lingers from the mists of time. It's a garden that confers such wonders and pleasures that it's transformative. It's the source of life: not only procreative but also regenerative and revivifying.

A man and woman in love who experience orgasm as an intense and intimate event feel themselves transported to a different dimension. They are showered by rays of the infinite. They become beings of light. The experience makes their very bodies luminous. The man who is patient with his wife, who is not a selfish lover, and who takes the time to stimulate her to this point will witness the flowering of her full femininity. He will see the infinite glowing from her countenance as she enters this transcendent realm.

> The man who is patient with his wife, who is not a selfish lover, and who takes the time to stimulate her to orgasmic ecstasy will witness the flowering of her full femininity.

Before his very eyes his wife becomes Eve, the supreme embodiment of all things feminine. She is all women, the feminine responding to the masculine.

He will watch her becoming luminous, like a supernova, her physical being transformed into pure energy. And in this primal moment he will love her and be drawn to her with an intensity that defies description.

Nature is based on cycles and rhythms. It is never static. And so, lovemaking also becomes like a tuning fork. It has a natural hum, a natural movement, an intuitive rhythm. Like a crystal that has an innate vibration, a man and woman in love develop a unified synchronicity. There is an underlying current of movement that underlies all of creation. The elements of a nucleus are in constant motion. Matter appears static but in truth is always in motion. And when a couple achieve spiritual transcendence in sex they begin to experience that deeper connection with the rhythm of nature and the cycle of life. Everything is alive, vibrant, and in motion.

Many mock the religious prohibition against masturbation. But the idea has depth. Reliving the pleasures of Eden must be through the medium of connection with another person. An orgasm can be experienced solo, but leaves a person feeling bereft in the aftermath because its purpose is to facilitate the spiritual orchestration of two halves in a moment of unadorned ecstasy that transcends the inherent separation of physicality. There is no comparison between a purely physical solitary experience and a transcendent spiritual experience leaving us emotionally bound to someone we love. One is a pleasure purely of the body; the other is a delight for the soul.

Speaking in such mind-blowing terms about the sexual experience, some people feel that it can or even should be artificially enhanced by the use of (usually illegal) drugs. When I lived in England, a woman whose sex life with her husband was moribund asked me whether they ought to use ecstasy, "E," to juice up their sex life. These were the go-go years of the artificial high in Great Britain, with giant raves and thousands of young people popping E. The woman had heard from her friends that sex on Ecstasy was ... well ... ecstasy. I told her that I am against taking drugs of any kind for the obvious reasons. But more importantly, orgasm is itself the greatest drug. The body can produce the most euphoric high – no external help needed. It raises you to the heights of pleasure and bliss. It makes you forget all cares and worries. It puts you in a place of utter relaxation. It makes you feel good all over. It offers a brief glimpse of paradise.

Those who think they need to get high to enjoy sex are

demonstrating the impotence of their own sexual experience. Sex is apparently such a dud that it requires an external
stimulant. On the contrary, orgasm is the ultimate drug, the
ultimate high, where the mind detonates, the body is pul-
verized, and the soul is set loose. Likewise a womanizer, or a
promiscuous woman who finds it difficult to sustain an intimate relationship, actually demonstrates the weakness of his
or her sexuality. For them sex is not powerful; it lacks depth.
Quantity demonstrates the absence of quality. A womanizer
can never really take enough pleasure in just one woman – he
needs more women because he fails to plumb the depths of
the one he has. A woman with intimacy issues similarly fails
to bond erotically to one man, becoming dependent on surface-deep sexual connections that are ultimately degrading
and sometimes even abusive.

Taking drugs or engaging in conquest of multiple partners
are both just forms of emotional avoidance. Some people
shy away from real intimacy, whether out of fear, laziness, or
ignorance of the true possibilities.

Two people can be physically engaged but emotionally
totally separate. Even intense physical gratification – if it stays
on the level of a physical experience and does not result in
emotional intimacy – completely misses the transformative
power of the intimate act. A deep spiritual communion, by
contrast, is bonding, healing, and transformative.

The test is what happens immediately after orgasm. Do
you both go to sleep on separate sides of the bed as if no
shared experience has happened, all desire dissipated, or do
you remain in each other's arms enjoying the strong bliss
and sense of togetherness that is fostered when two people
are transformed by an overwhelming intimate experience?

Without a passionate sex life, husband and wife experience deep loneliness even within marriage. I have counseled countless couples who have ceased having sex, which is another way of saying that they have ceased being intimate. Yes, they may have conversations. And deep conversations may engage the soul and the mind – they may tap into our higher spiritual capacity for distinct human contact. But mere talking leaves the body out of the equation. Separation remains palpable. Loneliness ensues. It's painful to see and hear these couples. To be lonely even while married is hell on earth.

It is not simple to go from a sexless marriage to a transcendent sexual experience. Sexless marriage leaves people feeling profoundly rejected. Emotional intimacy must be built. Hurts and disappointment must be overcome. But as a couple begins to draw closer and experience true intimacy, transcendence comes intuitively and automatically.

Ironically, many of the very things that often come between spouses and prevent them from being intimate with one another could be healed by the transcendent intimate experience. Everyday life entails pain and disappointment; many of us feel broken and cynical. Mystical intimacy with one's spouse can heal those broken pieces of our souls.

Limitation surrounds us at every turn. And it takes a lot to be drawn out. This is especially true as we get older and face so many of life's disappointments. We recoil from life's hurts. We learn to distrust the world. We become even more self-focused. We get more defensive. More barriers between us and the rest of the world are erected.

This happens especially in marriage. It is specifically the person who loves you the most who can wound you the most; many husbands and wives carry deep scar tissue in their relationships. In all this, physical intimacy is supposed to serve as a healing balm to counteract the wounds, the distance, and the pain. But this is especially true of orgasm. It is designed to serve as the supreme moment of extroversion, of coming out of one's shell, of sharing blissful pleasure with someone we love that raises us to a higher plane of existence. This is not a matter of forgetting one's problems but transcending them.

> I encouraged Fred, who came to me for counseling about depression, to stop popping pills and begin opening his heart. He and his wife were married for seventeen years and were having sex almost nightly. But what they had in passion they lacked in intimacy. Fred was desperate to open up to his wife emotionally, tell her about his feelings of failure, share with her his conviction that his life was passing him by. But he could not find the words. He was so closed, so utterly constrained. He could not discuss his pain. He could not share his loneliness. He needed to find a tool to open him up, make his soul less rigid and his spirit more malleable.
>
> So I encouraged him to use lovemaking with his wife as his method of communication. It had to stop being a purely physical interaction and become a spiritual conjoining of souls. "When you're making love to your wife," I told Fred, "I want you to look into her eyes as deeply as you possibly can. If she starts closing her eyes – whether out of ecstasy or concentration – prod her to open them up again. But don't lose that connection. And as the two of you approach that moment of sexual climax, focus on saying to her with your intense eye contact everything that is lacking in words.
>
> "At the moment of orgasm, as you experience the bodily sensations of pleasure, release all the pent-up pain, all the

suppressed loneliness. Obliterate all that divides you. Pull her as close as possible to you. Make it a moment of supreme connection. Don't focus the experience on yourself. Don't go deeper into yourself. Don't close your eyes and focus on the experience of physical bliss. When you do that, you're using sex as an escape. You're escaping pain, you're escaping loneliness. You're retreating into a world of pleasure that dulls pain. But it doesn't last. It doesn't change you. It doesn't take away loneliness and pain. In fact, it increases it. Because by the time you finish you're going to feel so let down. The reality of your everyday existence is going to be a disappointment. The pain will only increase.

"But if you use the power of sexual climax to come out of yourself, if you make it into a spiritual experience, if you utilize the elasticity of soul that it affords, then you'll connect with your wife in the deepest way. You'll even find that you actually feel the two of you are being joined as one. And no, this is not a substitute for conversation. You and your wife need to discuss your hurt and disappointments. You need to talk about the barriers that divide you and slowly remove them. But this definitely serves as a launching pad. It's a strong beginning. What you need is a rubber soul. Sexual orgasm is that moment of supreme spiritual elasticity."

In the moments of nonverbal communication that pass between husband and wife in a fully engaged intimate experience, they can communicate to each other whole books of emotion that would take days to utter.

Feeling loved and cherished is profoundly healing. But even more than that, the physical and spiritual union of husband and wife is an experience of transcendent union with the predestined other half of one's soul.

The Talmud weighs in on the Jewish concept of "*bashert*" – that is, the idea that one's romantic partner is destined from before one's birth: "Rabbi Judah says in the name of Rav: Forty days before a child is conceived, a *bat kol* [a voice from heaven] announces, 'The daughter of so-and-so is destined for so-and-so.'"[108] The Talmud reinforces the idea of the predestination of one's spouse with other quotations from Scripture: "Rav said in the name of Rabbi Reuven ben Itztroboli: We can prove from verses in the Torah, the Prophets, and the Writings, that the marriage of a man to his wife is predestined by God. From the Torah [when Abraham's manservant came to get Rebecca as a wife for Isaac]: 'Laban and Bethuel [Rebecca's brother and father] answered, "This is from the Lord"' (Genesis 24:50). From the Prophets [when Samson wanted to marry a Philistine woman]: 'His parents did not know that this was from the Lord' (Judges 14:4). And from the Writings: 'Houses and wealth are inherited from parents, but a prudent wife is from the Lord' (Proverbs 19:14)."[109]

Kabbalah refers to men and women as *plag nishmasa*, "half souls." The soul is said to be split into two parts: one half male and one half female. When the male and female join together in marriage, it is thus the reunification of the two halves of the soul.[110] The thirteenth-century Jewish sage Rabbi Shlomo ben Aderet, known by the acronym Rashba, explains that God first created man and woman together in one body and then split them apart, taking Eve from Adam's rib, so that when they unite they return to their original state of oneness.[111]

Maimonides goes so far as to say that they never left that state of oneness:

> ... Adam and Eve were two in some respects, and yet they remained one, according to the words "Bone of my bones,

and flesh of my flesh" (Genesis 2:23). The unity of the two is proved by the fact that both have the same name, for she is called *ishah* (woman), because she was taken out of *ish* (man), also by the words "And he shall cleave unto his wife, and they shall be one flesh" (Genesis 2:24).[112]

This is the ultimate potential of the intimate marital relationship: nothing less than the reunification of the other half of one's soul. Bone of my bones and flesh of my flesh. Transcendent wholeness.

A Working Model

We've been discussing some pretty heady stuff. Yet somehow in between the mind-blowing orgasms and the reunification of your souls, chances are you and your spouse will have to take some time out to go to work, cook dinner, put the kids to bed, and file taxes. How can we create a marriage that integrates the mundane realities of domesticity with the sublime rejuvenation of passion, for a marriage and a life that is alive and invigorated?

Once again let's turn to the wisdom of the Bible, which offers us a model for a synthesis of the elements of love and lust in a healthy fusion that makes for a durable and joyful marriage. I believe we can learn how to integrate the lust relationship and the love relationship in one coherent whole by studying the marriage of Jacob to his two wives Rachel and Leah.

When Jacob first meets Rachel, he seeks to impress her by moving a giant stone that is covering a well, then kisses her and breaks into tears. He then offers Laban, her father, seven years of work in return for Rachel's hand in marriage.

The years pass by so quickly that "it appeared in his eyes as if it were but days, so much did he long for her" (Genesis 29:20).

Jacob's love for Rachel is one of deep passion and yearning. It is love as covetousness and desire. It is the fieriest kind of romantic love. It is lust incarnate.

But it is also the most tragic kind of attraction. Romantic, passionate, lustful love that is unbalanced by partnership and intimacy nearly always ends badly, either because the fires die down or because the fire burns so brightly that it consumes both participants. Jacob feels in his bones that his passion for Rachel must end disastrously. Thus, he is drawn to kiss her, but he immediately weeps. He recognizes that in this imperfect world, perfect love is impossible to attain. He wants Rachel to be his soul mate, but he intuits that he is destined to lose her.

By contrast, he experiences none of the same passion for Leah. When he is fooled into marrying her, he accepts Leah as a partner and eventually as the mother of his children. But his yearning is for Rachel. Leah feels hated and names the first of her three children after her experiences of rejection from Jacob. The first is named Reuben (in Hebrew, *re'u, ben,* "See, a son"), "for she said, 'It is because the Lord has seen my misery. Surely my husband will love me now'" (Genesis 29:32). Simeon (in Hebrew, *shim-on,* "He heard my sorrow") is "Because the Lord heard that I am not loved, He gave me this one too" (Genesis 29:33). Levi is the son on whose account *yilaveh ishi elai,* "my husband will become attached to me" (Genesis 29:34). Only with the fourth son, Judah, which means "praise to God," do we begin to see a name that gives the child an intrinsic identity rather than one that relates instead to the relationship of his father to his mother.

For Jacob, Leah represents a maternal, practical partner

with whom he shares a life but has no passionate connection. They have intimacy but no intensity. They have a family but no fervor or fire. He is comfortable with her but does not lust after her. He loves her but does not long for her. He wishes to protect her but she is not the delight of his soul.

Yet Jacob knows in his heart that Leah, rather than Rachel, is destined to be his soul mate. She is destined to bear most of his children, share his life, and share eternity by being buried at his side at the Tomb of the Patriarchs in Hebron. Leah represents stability and order. She will be Jacob's anchor. She is his permanence, the woman who tethers him to family. Yet he will never make peace with love that is only functional and not romantic, stable but not passionate.

Rachel is playful, girlish, and evinces, at times, a short-sightedness that is often characteristic of women whom men desire mightily. She blames Jacob for her infertility. She can play the victim. She can also be callous about Jacob's love for her, knowing that because of its intensity she can afford to take it for granted. When Reuben brings mandrake flowers for his mother Leah, Rachel strikes a deal with Leah to exchange the flowers – said to be a fertility aid – for a conjugal night with Jacob. Rachel's longing for a child overshadows everything to the point that she does not see – as Leah does – the immense value of even one night of togetherness with her beloved. Unlike Jacob, who understands intuitively the tragic nature of passionate, romantic love, Rachel thinks they have endless time to be together. One night will make no difference. But Jacob knows the clock is ticking.

Women like Leah ultimately both triumph and suffer. In their stability they end up gaining the commitment of men who build families with them. But they suffer because they rarely feel the passionate desire of their husbands. They are partners to their husbands but not objects of lust. And a woman wants to be desired even more than she wants to be loved.

Jacob has two wives, each addressing different facets of his life. This is a phenomenon that seems as old as time itself. Many generals or kings in days of yore would have two women to fulfill two very different needs. The pedigreed wife bore children and ruled as a consort; the mistress brought passion and excitement. But our society rightly expects men who are accomplished in public life to be equally accomplished in marriage by finding both dimensions in one woman.

It is the amalgamation of both types of love that is meant to characterize the successful marriage. Not a man in a relationship with two women, but a man and woman whose marriage incorporates both dimensions. Husbands and wives are meant to have passion and practicality, fire and firmness, lust and love, desire and durability. *Rachel and Leah are meant to be one.*

The Jewish laws that are revealed with the giving of the Torah at Sinai will prescribe half of the month devoted to passion and sexual fire, and half of the month devoted to soulfulness and intimacy. The orchestration of the two is what makes a marriage whole. We are meant to be lovers and best friends, paramours and soul mates. Our wives should be our mistresses and our companions. We need the stability and practicality of love, but we also never wish to lose the passionate excitement of lust.

We have to learn how to amalgamate the two. And we have to internalize the fact that lust is not a nicety or an extra; it's not something that brings people together and then fades away into the sunset. Vibrant lust is critical to your marriage. Not only *can* it be kept alive, but it *must* be kept alive. Lust is not dirty. In marriage, it is positively kosher.

The synthesis of love and desire, of the passionate with the practical, of friendship with being lovers, is how kosher lust is created.

> The synthesis of love and desire, of the passionate with the practical, of friendship with being lovers, is how kosher lust is created.

So, practically speaking, how do we keep lust alive in the long term? How do we keep the steam within the marriage and focus on the exclusivity and primacy of that relationship so that erotic pressure builds in the right places – and only in the right places?

- Practice conversational intimacy. I'm a great believer that a couple's problems and issues are their problems (or their counselor or therapist's problems, where applicable). So many people – women especially – discuss intimate aspects of their marriages with friends. This is in truth something of a betrayal of your intimate relationship. Don't talk about your sex life with other people. Keep it in the bedroom, between the two of you, where it belongs. Accord your covenantal relationship the sanctity and dignity it deserves.

- Practice mental fidelity. If you allow your mind to become excited by others, that definitely dilutes your erotic dependence on your spouse. People masturbate, look at porn, flirt with strangers, think about other people, make love while thinking of others. This kind of mental roving directs your primary sexual organ (yes, your brain!) outside your marriage and diminishes the focus needed for true erotic intensity.

• Recognize the inherent power of natural sexual attraction, the incredible gravitation of the masculine to the feminine. In many ways, religious society has the potential to be the most sexual of all, because religious people don't believe that the relationship between a man and a woman is banal. We don't believe that just seeing a woman's beautiful form or hearing her mellifluous voice is nothing. We do not reduce women to prioritized erogenous zones. Rather, all of her body, if you are truly in love with her, can have an erotic quality. Think about the Beatles song "I Want to Hold Your Hand," which became the best-selling single in British history and is still named on all-time top hit lists the world over. Clearly there has to be something inherently erotic about holding a woman's hand for this song to have achieved such longevity. Remember Homer's *Odyssey*? Odysseus wants to hear the song of the incredibly seductive Sirens, thinking he will be able to resist their power, but their captivating female voices cause him to lose control and suffer temporary insanity. Men and women are naturally powerfully attracted to each other. Don't forget this.

• Don't put yourself in situations where the small embers of attraction to someone who is not your spouse grow to the point that you're going to have to suppress the feeling. Judaism is not a religion of repression or suppression. It acknowledges natural attraction and does not seek to suppress or repress it. Rather, what we try to do is ensure that attraction doesn't grow in inappropriate directions.

Don't put yourself into compromising situations where you're forced to suppress attraction to a third party. Don't minimize casual interactions that lead to erotic excitement that must later either be suppressed or it will just naturally grow. No matter what, if you're flirting with people you're not married to, you're diluting the erotic excitement from your spouse.

- Husbands: Make a conscious decision to derive erotic interest exclusively from your wife. For example, if you have a nanny in the home or if there is an attractive work colleague at the office, you know that you can have what seem to be casual exchanges but are, in fact, tiny erotic encounters. You can do all that and for you it seems totally innocent. But if you're fully honest with yourself you'll acknowledge that it's not completely without consequences. Everyone needs to have the erotic mind fed. When you diffuse your attentions all around, you're opening the lid of that pressure cooker and reducing the intensity in your marriage. Learn to train your erotic attention on your wife. Stare at her when she bends down and look for the outline of her undergarments. Steal flirtatious moments during the day to say something affectionate. Watch her interactions with other men and be reminded of her intrinsic attractiveness. They glimpse something in her that is about her womanhood. Noticing this helps you see her through the eyes of another to whom she is novel and new. When you keep your erotic attention focused on your wife, you're feeding your erotic attraction to her.

- Wives: Make a conscious decision to derive erotic interest exclusively from your husband. Women are just as excited by the erotic stimulation that strangers can provide and need to focus erotically on their husbands. It's a two-way street. This has become an age of great female flirtatiousness. Many women feel they are not getting the kind of attention they really want in their primary relationships, so they're seeking more and more of it outside of those relationships. Women, like men, get a great deal of erotic pleasure and excitement from third parties, through casual conversation, allowing men to flirt with them, showing their bodies to men knowing it's going to attract them. You need to understand that there's a consequence to this: flirting with other men causes a diminishment of primary attraction to your husband.

- Remember that unavailability is a prime condition of lust and use the times when you are apart to build your attraction. If one of you has to travel, send each other erotic notes, talk on the phone, and generally work yourselves into a frenzy that you will consummate when you are reunited. You can even do this during the workday (with the caveat that you have to be appropriate when at your workplace!).

- Don't treat your wife like a maid, mother, homemaker, and caretaker. When the practical trumps the erotic, your wife doesn't feel like a woman anymore. A husband has to bring out his wife's desire. Jewish values specify that a woman should be pleasured before her husband. Seeing his wife forfeit herself to wild erotic abandon creates desire in a husband too. It's a win-win.

- Don't treat your husband like nothing more than a workhorse provider. Men want to be valued for more than just the paycheck they bring home. Most men are very happy to provide for their families and even to check off items on a "honey-do" list, but a man wants to feel like more than just a cash machine and a handyman to his wife. He needs to feel valued for who he is and not just for what he can do.

• Realize that the little things are not little. We tend to think that as long as spouses are not committing technical infidelity or engaging in extremely compromising behavior, then anything goes. But it's a choice you're making: Where are you going to invest your erotic energy? Where you invest, that's where you will see returns.

Finally, I want to leave you with this thought: *it matters.* When the *New York Times* published its important article on the problem of the loss of female desire in long-term relationships (Daniel Bergner, "Unexcited? There May Be a Pill for That," May 22, 2013), I was struck by the number of reader comments that expressed some form of the message "The truth is that sex is not all that important." If you've lost your desire, say these readers, who cares? Sex isn't the be-all and end-all, and if it fades as life goes on, then we should just embrace the new warm and fuzzy companionable stage of our marriages.

One woman who loved her husband deeply but whose marriage had become entirely platonic told me that sex was like frozen yogurt. It's an individual taste. Some people love it. Others can do without it.

I could not disagree more.

"Do not go gentle into that good night," wrote the Welsh poet Dylan Thomas in 1951. "Rage, rage against the dying of the light."

In Jewish law, the marital act, the highest form of intimacy, is formally a husband's obligation to his wife, included in the *ketubah*, the Jewish wedding contract. I once heard a story about an elderly man who felt that with all his aches and pains, it was time to let his intimate relationship with his wife go. He asked her permission to be released from his obligation to her in this area and she granted it. Then he went to his rabbi to formally request to be absolved from his conjugal obligation to his wife, being sure to tell the rabbi that his wife had already given her consent. The rabbi shook his head sadly. "The fact that your wife is willing to end your physical relationship proves to me that you have never fulfilled this commandment even once in your life. If you had, she would never have been willing to give it up."

How many of us are similarly missing the point? Do we realize the power of the intimate marital relationship? Do we even know what we're missing?

I hope that in the pages of this book I have convinced you that your sexual and erotic relationship with your spouse is holy, necessary, and worth fighting for. Yes, we must all have the Jacob-Leah relationship: we must be stable, responsible people who take care of our domestic obligations, care for our children if we have been granted that privilege, and together uphold our values and contribute to our communities. But how will we ever have the vital energy to fulfill all these obligations if we are not also fueled by the passion of the Jacob-Rachel relationship?

To embrace Eros is to embrace life itself. To embrace it in sanctity within our marriages is to honor our spouses, our own souls, and God.

So go on: live, love, and lust.

Acknowledgments

This book has been the project of several years, with many stops and starts. Lust and the erotic mind are some of the most difficult subjects in the world to truly understand, and as I started to write the book I realized that I needed greater clarity. I therefore waited to finish the writing until I had researched the subject more, given more lectures, written and received feedback on more articles, and counseled more troubled marriages, so I could deepen my insight. Therefore, the first thank you that has to be given in this book is to all the audiences who helped me refine these concepts as I lectured on the subject of kosher lust around the world over the last five years, as well as to the many married couples who trusted in me to help and better their relationships and through the counseling of whom I came to understand desire, lust, and eroticism much more profoundly.

As to individuals, I want to first thank the people at Gefen who have now published three of my books. Ilan Greenfield, Gefen's publisher, as well as his partner, Michael Fischberger, have believed fully in my books and have disseminated my ideas throughout the world, for which I am deeply grateful. Lynn Douek, the projects coordinator, shepherded the book through production with efficiency and grace.

Kezia Raffel Pride has now edited two of my books, only

this time she put a huge amount of time into reworking the material into more structured chapters and taking so many of my loose thoughts and giving them form and definition. I am absolutely grateful to her. Kezia is one of the most brilliant editors I have ever worked with, and much more importantly, she is a woman of the highest morality, integrity, wisdom, and insight.

I of course want to thank my children, who just through everyday discussions about life deepen my understanding of human nature. My wife and I, while I was writing this book, had the great pleasure of becoming grandparents to little Mirele. I want to thank my son-in-law, Arik, my eldest daughter Mushki, my daughters Chana, Shterny, Shaina, Baba, and Cheftziba, and my sons Mendy, Yosef, and David Chaim, for being true inspirations to me in all matters of life and work. Children are the greatest joy and God's most precious blessing.

I want to thank my wife Debbie, my soul mate and inspiration. She is to me the living embodiment of femininity and ladylike dignity and has taught me, through her very being, about the beauty of marriage, the warmth of human relationships, and the transcendent bond that connects a man and a woman.

Above all else, I am grateful to God Almighty for the blessings He has given me and my wife and my children, and for my ability to bring universal Jewish wisdom and values to the public. I hope this book will make a difference in your relationship and solidify and bring sparks to your marriage.

Rabbi Shmuley Boteach
October 2013
United States of America

Notes

1. This is a difficult statistic to nail down. Simplistically, it's based on the fact that each year approximately half as many people divorce as marry (See "National Marriage and Divorce Rate Trends," Centers for Disease Control and Prevention, National Vital Statistics System, http://www. cdc.gov/nchs/nvss/marriage_divorce_tables.htm). Of course, the divorces that take place in a given year are mostly not the same couples who married that year, so the correlation is not clear. Nevertheless, following discussions with demography experts and a detailed analysis of available data, the New Jersey watchdog site Politifact.com concluded that "the overall probability of marriages now ending in divorce falls between 40 percent and 50 percent" (http://www.politifact.com/ new-jersey/statements/2012/feb/20/stephen-sweeney/steve-sweeney-claims-more-two-thirds-marriages-end/).

2. Overall life expectancy in the United States is 78.49 years (CIA World Factbook, 2012 estimates, https://www.cia.gov/library/publications/ the-world-factbook/geos/us.html). US life expectancy a hundred years earlier, in 1912, was just 53.5 years (National Vital Statistics Reports, vol. 61, no. 3, September 24, 2012, http://www.cdc.gov/nchs/data/nvsr/ nvsr61/nvsr61_03.pdf).

3. Just 48 percent of American households were married couples in 2010, according to census data analyzed by the Brookings Institution. Sabrina Tavernise, "Married Couples Are No Longer a Majority, Census Finds," *New York Times*, May 26, 2011.

4. The total percentage of widowed, divorced, separated, or never married women over age eighteen in the United States is 47.9 percent. Unmarried men in the same categories total 44.8 percent. US Census Bureau, "America's Families and Living Arrangements: 2011," Table A1, http:// www.census.gov/population/www/socdemo/hh-fam/cps2011.html.

5. See for example Alexandra Brewis and Mary Meyer, "Marital Coitus across the Life Course," *Journal of Biosocial Science* 37, no. 4 (2005): 499–518, which analyzed Demographic and Health Survey data in nineteen nations around the world and found decline in frequency of marital intimacy from early in the life course to late in the life course ranging from 20.6 percent (in Bangladesh) to 74 percent (in the Philippines). Vaughn Call, Susan Sprecher, and Pepper Schwartz, in their study "The Incidence and Frequency of Marital Sex in a National Sample," *Journal*

of Marriage and Family 57, no. 3 (August 1995), found that on average, newlywed couples in the US are intimate three times per week, declining in early middle age to one and a half to two times per week, and over age fifty once a week or less.

6. Pew Research Center, "Marriage Is Obsolete," January 6, 2011, http://www.pewresearch.org/daily-number/marriage-is-obsolete/.

7. Pew Research Center analysis of Decennial Census (1960–2000) and American Community Survey Data (2008, 2010), Integrated Public Use Microdata Series.

8. US Census Bureau, 1970 Census, 2000 Census, and 2008 American Community Survey, cited in Linda A. Jacobsen and Mark Mather, "U.S. Economic and Social Trends since 2000," *Population Bulletin* 65, no. 1 (February 2010): 9, http://www.prb.org/Articles/2010/usmarriage-decline.aspx.

9. In 2009, the median duration of both first and second marriages that ended in divorce was eight years. Table 8, Median Duration of Marriages for People 15 Years and Over by Sex, Race, and Hispanic Origin: 2009, in Rose M. Kreider and Renee Ellis, "Number, Timing, and Duration of Marriages and Divorces: 2009," *Current Population Reports* P70-125 (Washington, DC: US Census Bureau, 2011).

10. "Median Age at First Marriage, 1960–2011," in D'Vera Cohn, Jeffrey Passel, Wendy Wang, and Gretchen Livingston, "Barely Half of U.S. Adults Are Married – A Record Low," Pew Research Social and Demographic Trends, December 14, 2011, http://www.pewsocialtrends.org/2011/12/14/barely-half-of-u-s-adults-are-married-a-record-low/#fn-10398-1.

11. Based on figures in US Census Bureau, Current Population Survey, 2011 Annual Social and Economic Supplement, Table A1 all races, http://www.census.gov/population/www/socdemo/hh-fam/cps2011.html.

12. The rate in 2008 was 41 percent. Mark Mather and Diana Lavery, "In U.S., Proportion Married at Lowest Recorded Levels," Population Reference Bureau, September 2010, www.prb.org/Articles/2010/usmarriagedecline.aspx. By 2010 it had remained constant at 40.8 percent. Mary Seaborn, "Marriage in America: The Fraying Knot," *The Economist*, January 12, 2013.

13. Based on analysis of data from the National Center for Health Statistics by Child Trends. Jason DeParle and Sabrina Tavernise, "For Women Under 30, Most Births Occur Outside Marriage," *New York Times*, February 17, 2012.

14. The marriage rate in the Nordic countries in 2011 ranged from a low of 4.0 marriages per thousand people in the Åland Islands to a high of 5.3 in Finland. *Nordic Statistical Yearbook 2012*, http://www.norden.org/en/publications/publikationer/2012-001. By contrast, in 2009, 2010, and 2011 the US registered 6.8 marriages per thousand people. National Marriage and Divorce Rate Trends, National Vital Statistics System, http://www.cdc.gov/nchs/nvss/marriage_divorce_tables.htm.

15. Trine Anker, quoted in Noelle Knox, "Nordic Family Ties Don't Mean Tying the Knot," *USA Today*, December 15, 2004.

16. In 2010 South American countries logged marriage rates as low as 3.2 (Uruguay), 3.0 (Argentina), 2.8 (Peru), and 2.5 (French Guiana). United Nations Statistics Division, Marriages and Crude Marriage Rates, http://unstats.un.org/unsd/demographic/products/dyb/dyb2011/Table23.pdf.

17. "The State of Our Unions: Marriage in America 2012," University of Virginia National Marriage Project, http://nationalmarriageproject.org/wp-content/uploads/2012/12/SOOU2012.pdf.

18. Ibid.

19. Mindy E. Scott, Erin Schelar, Jennifer Manlove, and Carol Cui, "Young Adult Attitudes about Relationships and Marriage: Times May Have Changed, but Expectations Remain High," Child Trends Research Brief, Publication #2009-30, July 2009, http://www.childtrends.org/Files//Child_Trends-2009_07_08_RB_YoungAdultAttitudes.pdf.

20. Shirley P. Glass and Thomas L. Wright, "Sex Differences in Type of Extramarital Involvement and Marital Dissatisfaction," *Sex Roles* 12, no. 9–10 (May 1985): 1101–1120.

21. Eros is typically understood to mean desire, and usually specifically sexual desire. But, as James and Evelyn Whitehead explain in their book *Holy Eros: Recovering the Passion of God* (Maryknoll, NY: Orbis Books, 2009), "Psychologists and theologians today are restoring *eros's* battered reputation. By drawing on the word's earliest meanings, they are reclaiming *eros* as the fundamental vitality of the human person. This broader meaning encompasses sexual arousal and more. *Eros* is ardent desire. Rooted in our bodies, *eros* links us passionately to life" (p. 53).

22. Studies estimate that 15 to 20 percent of couples live in a "sexless marriage," defined as a marriage in which intimate marital relationships are limited to ten times per year or less. Kathleen Deveny, "No Sex, Please, We're Married," *Newsweek*, June 30, 2003. According to the 2005 National Opinion Research Center General Social Survey, about one

in five married couples are in sexless marriages, but the figure is worse in "long-term" marriages (defined by the survey as having lasted two years or more): one in every three of these couples reported they are intimate less than ten times per year!

23. The National Opinion Research Center General Social Survey for 2005 reported that married couples have sex sixty-six times a year, or slightly more often than once a week.

24. *The Life and Work of Sigmund Freud*, ed. Ernest Jones, vol. 2 (New York: Basic Books, 1955), part 3, chapter 16, p. 421.

25. Midrash on Proverbs 31:10.

26. "Seventeenth-century French physician Jacques Ferrand...argued that lovesickness in all its manifestations was more likely to affect women because they were less rational, more 'maniacal,' and more libidinous in their love [than men]." Jacques Ferrand, *A Treatise on Lovesickness*, 1623, ed. and trans. Donald A. Beecher and Massimo Ciavolella (Syracuse: Syracuse University Press, 1990), 311, discussed in Carol Groneman, "Nymphomania: The Historical Construction of Female Sexuality," *Signs: Journal of Women in Culture and Society* 19, no. 2 (winter 1994): 337–67.

27. *Malleus Maleficarum*, 1486, cited and translated in *Witchcraft in Europe 1100–1700: A Documentary History*, ed. Alan C. Kors and Edward Peters (Philadelphia: University of Philadelphia Press, 1972), 127.

28. "Some Thoughts Concerning the Stage in a Letter to a Lady" (1704), cited in Daryl Ogden, *The Language of the Eyes: Science, Sexuality, and Female Vision in English Literature and Culture, 1690–1927* (Albany: State University of New York Press, 2005), 24.

29. John and Robin Haller, *The Physician and Sexuality in Victorian America* (Urbana: University of Illinois Press, 1974), discussed in Estelle B. Freedman and John D'Emilio, "Problems Encountered in Writing the History of Sexuality: Sources, Theory and Interpretation," *Journal of Sex Research* 27, no. 4 (November 1990): 482.

30. Groneman, "Nymphomania," 337–67.

31. Her studies include M.L. Chivers, M.C. Seto, et al., "Agreement of Genital and Subjective Measures of Sexual Arousal in Men and Women: A Meta-Analysis," *Archives of Sexual Behavior* 39 (2010): 5–56.

32. Daniel Bergner, *What Do Women Want? Adventures in the Science of Female Desire* (New York: Ecco, 2013), 13.

33. Ibid., 61–63.

34. Irene Tsapelas, Helen E. Fisher, and Arthur Aron, "Infidelity: When, Where, Why," in William R. Cupach and Brian H. Spitzberg, *The Dark*

Side of Close Relationships II (New York: Routledge, 2010), 175–96. To be fair, most recent studies find more modest rates of marital infidelity, on the order of 20–40 percent of men and 20–25 percent of women. See for example A. Greeley, "Marital Infidelity," *Society* 31 (1994): 9–13 and Melissa Ann Tafoya and Brian H. Spitzberg, "The Dark Side of Infidelity: Its Nature, Prevalence, and Communicative Functions," in Brian H. Spitzberg and William R. Cupach, eds., *The Dark Side of Interpersonal Communication*, 2nd ed. (Mahwah, NJ: Lawrence Erlbaum Associates, 2007), 201–42.

35. See for example Michael W. Wiederman, "Extramarital Sex: Prevalence and Correlates in a National Survey," *Journal of Sex Research* 34, no. 2 (spring 1997): 167–74. This study found no difference between male and female levels of infidelity in respondents under age 40.

36. In 2009–2010 in the United States, women received 62 percent of all associate's degrees, 57.4 percent of all bachelor's degrees, 62.6 percent of all master's degrees, and 53.3 percent of all doctoral degrees (including PhDs, MDs, DDS, and law degrees). "The Condition of Education 2012 (NCES 2012-045)," Table A-47-2, US Department of Education, National Center for Education Statistics. In 2013, for the first time ever, more women than men received PhDs in the sciences in all three major Israeli universities (Tel Aviv University, the Hebrew University, and Bar-Ilan University). Dudi Goldman, "More Doctorates to Women Than Men in Israeli Universities in 2013," Ynet, June 4, 2013.

37. A 2009 study concluded that "U.S. girls now perform as well as boys on standardized mathematics tests at all grade levels." Janet S. Hyde, Janet E. Mertz, and Randy Schekman, "Gender, Culture, and Mathematics Performance," *Proceedings of the National Academy of Sciences of the United States of America* 106, no. 22 (June 2, 2009): 8801–8807. Nevertheless it should be noted that boys still score an average thirty points higher on the SAT math test than girls. "The SAT® Report on College and Career Readiness: 2012," http://media.collegeboard.com/digitalServices/pdf/research/TotalGroup-2012.pdf.

38. Madeleine Albright (1997–2001), Condoleezza Rice (2005–2009), and Hilary Rodham Clinton (2009–2013).

39. Margaret F. Brinig and Douglas W. Allen, "'These Boots Are Made for Walking': Why Most Divorce Filers Are Women," *American Law and Economics Review* 2, no. 1 (spring 2000): 126–69.

40. Katie Roiphe, "Spanking Goes Mainstream," *Newsweek*, April 16, 2012.

41. Allison Pearson, "Why Multi-Tasking Mothers Yearn for Fifty Shades of Grey," *Telegraph*, July 18, 2012.
42. Bergner, *What Do Women Want?*, 78.
43. "Husbands Who Extinguish Their Wives' Libidos," *Huffington Post*, February 17, 2013.
44. Bergner, *What Do Women Want?*, 77.
45. Ibid., 64.
46. S. Andrea Miller and E. Sandra Byers, "Actual and Desired Duration of Foreplay and Intercourse: Discordance and Misperceptions within Heterosexual Couples," *Journal of Sex Research* 41 (2004): 304. The seven-minute average found by Miller and Byers is actually an improvement, as in Kinsey's research in the 1940s and '50s, three-quarters of men self-reported that intercourse lasted under two minutes. Alfred C. Kinsey, Wardell B. Pomeroy, Clyde E. Martin, and Paul H. Gebhard, *Sexual Behavior in the Human Female* (Philadelphia: Saunders, 1953).
47. See Dalma Heyn, *The Erotic Silence of the American Wife* (New York: Plume, 1997), 14–15.
48. "[T]he creator had gradually been seduced by his creature." Henri Troyat, *Tolstoy* (New York: Doubleday and Company, 1967), 359. See Troyat's full analysis of Tolstoy's attitude toward Anna on pages 359–61.
49. Judith A. Levy, "Sex and Sexuality in Later Life Stages," in *Sexuality across the Life Course*, ed. Alice S. Rossi (Chicago: University of Chicago Press, 1994), 300. This book also cites Masters and Johnson's 1966 finding that "women who have sex once a month or less [the definition of "sexless marriage" which we discussed in chapter 1] may experience discomfort at penetration." Ibid.
50. "Prolonged sexual abstinence may itself suppress desire." Donald W. Black and Nancy C. Andreasen, *Introductory Textbook of Psychiatry* (Arlington, VA: American Psychiatric Publishing, 2011), 324.
51. "Women who remain sexually active...are less likely to have problems with vaginal dryness or lack of lubrication than women who undergo prolonged periods of abstinence." Richard D. McAnulty and Mary Michele Burnette, *Sex and Sexuality*, vol. 2, *Sexual Function and Dysfunction* (Westport, CT: Greenwood Publishing, 2006), 199. These authors also evoke Masters and Johnson's 1966 findings and posit that the famous researchers, among others, would support the "use it or lose it" approach. Ibid.
52. Pamela Madsen, "Sex: The More You Have – The More You Want?" *Psychology Today*, March 22, 2011.

53. The scenario of a bored, depressed, irritable, and dependent retired husband has become so prevalent, it led a Boise physician to coin the term "Retired Husband Syndrome" to describe the resulting stress-related illnesses among the retirees' wives. Charles Clifford Johnson, MD, "The Retired Husband Syndrome," *Western Journal of Medicine* 141 (October 1984): 542–45.
54. "Women report[ed] less negative reactions to unemployment than men." Richard E. Lucas, et al., "Unemployment Alters the Set Point for Life Satisfaction," *Psychological Science* 15, no. 1 (January 2004): 10.
55. "John Edwards, Former Democratic Presidential Candidate, Admits to Affair," *New York Times*, August 8, 2008.
56. Shirley P. Glass and Thomas L. Wright, "Sex Differences in Type of Extramarital Involvement and Marital Dissatisfaction," *Sex Roles* 12, no. 9–10 (May 1985): 1101–20.
57. Lewis Yablonsky, *The Extra-Sex Factor* (Bloomington, IN: iUniverse, 2009), 284.
58. M. Gary Neuman, *The Truth about Cheating: Why Men Stray and What You Can Do to Prevent It* (Hoboken, NJ: John Wiley and Sons, 2008).
59. Ibid.
60. Cited in Andrea Canning, "Rep. Anthony Weiner's Sexting Scandal: Why Did He Do It?" *ABC News*, June 6, 2011.
61. Vaughn R. Steele, Cameron Staley, Timothy Fong, Nicole Prause, "Sexual Desire, Not Hypersexuality, Is Related to Neurophysiological Responses Elicited by Sexual Images," *Socioaffective Neuroscience and Psychology* 3 (2013).
62. Neuman, *The Truth about Cheating*.
63. Loss of libido is especially problematic with the most commonly prescribed antidepressants, selective serotonin reuptake inhibitors (SSRIs), such as fluoxetine (Prozac), sertraline (Zoloft), paroxetine (Paxil), fluvoxamine (Luvox), citalopram (Celexa), and escitalopram (Lexapro). These SSRIs, as well as two other antidepressants called venlafaxine (Effexor) and clomipramine (Anafranil), have long been known to suppress libido and to cause associated problems with sexual function. See for example A.L. Montejo, et al., "Incidence of Sexual Dysfunction Associated with Antidepressant Agents: A Prospective Multicenter Study of 1022 Outpatients; Spanish Working Group for the Study of Psychotropic-Related Sexual Dysfunction," *Journal of Clinical Psychiatry* 62, suppl. 3 (2001): 10–21. Eleven percent of Americans aged 12 years and over take antidepressant medication, according to the Centers for

Disease Control and Prevention. Laura A. Pratt, Ph.D., et al., "Antidepressant Use in Persons Aged 12 and Over: United States, 2005–2008," National Center for Health Statistics Data Brief no. 76, October 2011.

64. David Nasaw, *The Chief: The Life of William Randolph Hearst* (New York: Mariner Books, 2001), 354.

65. Sigmund Freud, address to the Vienna B'nai B'rith, *The Standard Edition of the Complete Psychological Works of Sigmund Freud*, trans. and ed. James Strachey (London: Hogarth, 1956–1974), 20: 273–74.

66. Emily M. Brown, *Patterns of Infidelity and Their Treatment* (New York: Brunner-Routledge, 2001), 218.

67. Cited in Louise Lague, "From Mistress to Wife: Now What?" *Ladies' Home Journal* (2003), http://www.lhj.com/relationships/marriage/basics/from-mistress-to-wife-now-what/?page=4.

68. Of these, 12 percent had married twice and 3 percent had married three or more times. Rose M. Kreider and Renee Ellis, "Number, Timing, and Duration of Marriages and Divorces: 2009," *Current Population Reports* P70-125 (Washington, DC: US Census Bureau, 2011).

69. Cited in Josiah Hotchkiss Gilbert, *Dictionary of Burning Words of Brilliant Writers: A Cyclopaedia of Quotations from the Literature of All Ages* (1895), 392.

70. Cited in Daniel Povinelli and Nicholas G. Ballew, *World without Weight: Perspectives on an Alien Mind* (Oxford, UK: Oxford University Press, 2012), xv.

71. *The World of George Jean Nathan: Essays, Reviews, and Commentary* (New York: Applause, 1998), 161.

72. David Jackson, "Obama Praises Calif. AG's Looks," *USA Today*, April 4, 2013.

73. Ruben Navarrette Jr., "Obama's 'Best-Looking' Remark Was Sexist," CNN, April 7, 2013.

74. Josh Richman, "Obama Calls Comment on Kamala Harris a 'Teaching Moment,'" *Silicon Valley Mercury News*, April 17, 2013.

75. John Ziegler, "The Myth of Sarah Palin's Stupidity," *Daily Caller*, May 23, 2011.

76. Jill Lawrence, "Palin: Don't Hate Her Because She's Beautiful," *Politics Daily*, June 30, 2009.

77. Joan Walsh, "Kamala Harris Deserves Better," *Salon*, April 5, 2013.

78. See for example Deborah Tannen, *You Just Don't Understand! Men and Women in Conversation* (New York: Morrow, 1990); Anne Moir and David Jessel, *Brain Sex: The Real Difference between Men and Women*

(New York: Carol Publishing Group, 1991); and Deborah Blum, *Sex on the Brain: The Biological Differences between Men and Women* (New York: Penguin, 1998).

79. Aristotle, *Nicomachean Ethics* I:5, translated by W.D. Ross.
80. Numbered Exodus 20:17 and Deutoronomy 5:21 in Christian Bibles.
81. Rashi, commentary on Exodus 38:8.
82. Talmud *Shabbat* 63a.
83. Deuteronomy 13:5 (numbered 13:4 in Christian Bibles), from the Jewish Publication Society's 1917 translation.
84. From the Jewish Publication Society's 1917 translation.
85. See the Jewish Publication Society's 1917 translation: "Behold now, I know that thou art a fair woman to look upon" (based on King James, which is identical, as are the American Standard, the 1599 Geneva Bible, and others); the New American Standard Bible updates to "See now, I know that you are a beautiful woman"; NIV, together with other editions, modernizes and leaves out both *hinei* and *na*, rendering: "I know what a beautiful woman you are."
86. Rashi's commentary on Genesis 12:11, citing Midrash Tanhuma 5.
87. My translation.
88. Translation of the ArtScroll Sapirstein Edition *The Torah: With Rashi's Commentary Translated, Annotated, and Elucidated* (New York: Mesorah Publications, 1995). Compare King James: "Isaac was sporting with Rebekah his wife" (The Jewish Publication Society's 1917 version and the American Standard Version follow King James). The New International Version hints at the intended meaning by euphemistically translating, "Isaac [was] caressing his wife Rebekah."
89. Rashi's commentary on Genesis 24:65.
90. The twins' age at the time of the incident of the selling of the lentils is traditionally established by Rashi's explanation, in his commentary on Genesis 25:30, that Jacob had prepared these lentils as mourners' food, as the twins' grandfather Abraham had died that day. We know from Genesis 25:7 that Abraham lived to be 175 years old. And we know from Genesis 21:5 that Abraham was 100 years old when Isaac was born. Isaac was therefore 75 years old when his father Abraham died, and the twins, born when Isaac was 60 (Genesis 25:26), were 15.
91. Rashi, commentary on Genesis 29:11.
92. My translation.
93. See for example UCLA professor Linda J. Sax's book detailing her study of 17,000 college students, showing that girls thrive in single-sex educa-

tional environments: *The Gender Gap in College: Maximizing the Developmental Potential of Women and Men* (Hoboken, NJ: Jossey-Bass, 2008).

94. Allan Bloom, *The Closing of the American Mind: How Higher Education Has Failed Democracy and Impoverished the Souls of Today's Students* (New York: Simon and Schuster, 1987), 107.

95. Cited in Kate Taylor, "Sex on Campus: She Can Play That Game, Too," *New York Times*, July 12, 2013.

96. Ibid.

97. Daniel Bergner, "Unexcited? There May Be a Pill for That," *New York Times*, May 22, 2013.

98. Note that the husband's warning to his wife is inferred from the wording of the text, as the classic commentator Rashi explains. My description of this highly complex episode includes a number of such interpretations and clarifications, which you will not see if you read a standard English Bible text. For the full commentary by Rashi, see for example the Sapirstein edition Torah with Rashi's commentary translated, annotated, and elucidated (New York: ArtScroll/Mesorah, 1997).

99. Maimonides, *Hilkhot Sotah* 2:1.

100. Note however that if her husband has at any time himself been unfaithful, the waters will not have the power to harm her even if she is in fact guilty. Maimonides, *Hilkhot Sotah* 2:8, 3:17–19.

101. Rashi, Numbers 5:31.

102. Numbered Exodus 20:1–17 and Deuteronomy 5:4–21 in Christian Bibles.

103. Rashi, Numbers 5:31. Halachic commentators actually go so far as to say that in contemporary times, when we no longer have a Temple and therefore do not have access to the bitter waters and cannot conduct this test, a man must be careful not to label his wife as a suspected adulteress because she will henceforth become forbidden to him, without remedy, and he will be obliged to divorce her. Yad, *Sotah* 1.

104. Audrey Nelson, PhD, and Claire Damken Brown, PhD, *The Gender Communication Handbook: Conquering Conversational Collisions between Men and Women* (Hoboken, NJ: Wiley, 2012), 44.

105. See for example Jessica L. Tracy and Alec T. Beall, "Happy Guys Finish Last: The Impact of Emotion Expressions on Sexual Attraction," *Emotion* (May 23, 2011), which showed brooding or proud men were rated as more attractive by women than men who appeared happy. Another study divided men into two groups, one of which was treated to a heavy application of a high-end deodorant spray, and then photographed them. When shown the photographs, women rated the deodorant-sprayed

men as more attractive. Since the women obviously could not smell the deodorant, the greater attractiveness of these men must have stemmed from their own heightened confidence. S. Craig Roberts, et al., "Manipulation of Body Odour Alters Men's Self-Confidence and Judgments of Their Visual Attractiveness by Women," *International Journal of Cosmetic Science* 31, no. 1 (February 2009): 47–54.

106. The number of women who reported "always" climaxing during intercourse in a sampling of sixteen different surveys ranged from 6 percent to 51 percent, with the mean value being 25.3 percent. Elisabeth Anne Lloyd, *The Case of the Female Orgasm: Bias in the Science of Evolution* (Cambridge, MA: Harvard University Press, 2005), 27.

107. My translation. Psalms 45:13 in Christian Bibles, numbered 45:14 in the Jewish Tanakh.

108. Talmud *Sotah* 2a.

109. Talmud *Moed Katan* 18b.

110. This is explained by Nachmanides in his *Emunah u'Bitachon*, chapter 24.

111. Rashba, *Teshuvot* 1:60.

112. Moses Maimonides, *Guide for the Perplexed*, trans. M. Friedlander, PhD, 2d ed. (London: Routledge and Kegan Paul Ltd., 1904), 2:30.